Surgery of Genitourinary Pelvic Tumors

An Anatomic Atlas

J. Edson Pontes, M.D.

Wayne State University
School of Medicine
Detroit, Michigan

William Loechel

Medical Artist

WILEY-LISS

A JOHN WILEY & SONS, INC., PUBLICATION
New York • Chichester • Brisbane • Toronto • Singapore

Address All Inquiries to the Publisher
Wiley-Liss, Inc., 605 Third Avenue, New York, NY 10158-0012

© 1993 Wiley-Liss, Inc.

Printed in the United States of America

While the authors, editor, and publisher believe that drug selection and dosage and the specification and usage of equipment and devices, as set forth in this book, are in accord with current recommendations and practice at the time of publication, they accept no legal responsibility for any errors or omissions, and make no warranty, express or implied, with respect to material contained herein. In view of ongoing research, equipment modifications, changes in governmental regulations and the constant flow of information relating to drug therapy, drug reactions, and the use of equipment and devices, the reader is urged to review and evaluate the information provided in the package insert or instructions for each drug, piece of equipment, or device for, among other things, any changes in the instructions or indication of dosage or usage and for added warnings and precautions.

Library of Congress Cataloging-in-Publication Data

Pontes, J. Edson.
    Surgery of genitourinary pelvic tumors: an anatomic atlas / J.
Edson Pontes; William Loechel, illustrations.
      p. cm.
    Includes index.
    ISBN 0-471-58831-8
    1. Genitourinary organs—Tumors—Surgery—Atlases.
2. Genitourinary organs—Cancer—Surgery—Atlases. 3. Anatomy,
Surgical and topographical—Atlases.
    [DNLM: 1. Urogenital Neoplasms—surgery—atlases. WJ 17 P814s
1993]
RD670.P65 1993
616.99'26059—dc20
DNLM/DLC
for Library of Congress   93-17856

The text of this book is printed on acid-free paper.

Contents

Preface   vii

1   Anatomy of the Pelvis   1

The Bony Pelvis   2

Muscles and Ligaments   4

Nerves and Plexuses   10

The Autonomic Nervous System   10

The Vascular System   12

Urogenital Organs in the Pelvis   14

The Pelvic Ureter   14

The Urinary Bladder   14

The Prostate   16

2   Surgery of the Bladder and Lower Ureter   17

Partial Cystectomy   18

Tumor in a Diverticulum   22

*Partial Cystectomy for Tumors Located Near
the Ureteral Orifice*   24

Distal Ureterectomy–Ureteral Reimplant   26

Pelvic Lymphadenectomy   28

Pelvic Lymphadenectomy in Bladder Cancer   28

Radical Cystectomy   30

Radical Cystectomy in Women   38

3   Urinary Diversion   39

Noncontinent Urinary Diversion   40

Bricker Ureteroileal Anastomosis   42

Wallace Ureteroileal Anastomosis   44
Continent Urinary Diversion to the Skin   46
Continent Urinary Diversion to the Urethra   52
LeBag Continent Urinary Diversion   52
W Pouch with Absorbable Staple Anastomosis   54

4   Operations for Urinary Fistulas   59
Vesicovaginal Fistulas   60
Vaginal Repair of Vesicovaginal Fistulas   60
Abdominal Repair of Vesicovaginal Fistulas   62
Vesicoenteric Fistulas   66
The Use of the Omentum Flap   70

5   Radical Prostatectomy   73

6   Surgery for Penile and Urethral Cancers   81
Penile and Urethral Cancers   82
Superficial Inguinal Node Dissection   88
*Surgery for Local Tumor Recurrence of
the Superficial Inguinal Region*   92
Tensor Fasciae Latae Flap   94
Rectus Abdominis Flap   96

7   Reconstruction of the Urinary Tract during
Surgery for Rectal Tumors   101

8   Pelvic Sarcomas   109

References   117

Index   119

Preface

This atlas is intended to provide a quick reference for those who are embarking on urological oncologic procedures in the pelvis. The author has attempted to present surgical approaches with simplicity and uniformity.

The book opens with detailed review of the anatomy of the pelvis, integrating the bony structures and ligaments, muscles, blood vessels and lymphatics, nerves and plexuses, and urogenital organs in the pelvis. This should give the reader a solid background for the rest of the book.

In subsequent chapters, each operative procedure is illustrated with step-by-step drawings that are augmented on the facing page by concise descriptions of rationale, surgical technique, and pitfalls.

Specific procedures covered in the atlas include partial and radical cystectomy, distal ureterectomy, urinary diversion, repair of vesico-vaginal and vesicoenteric fistulas, radical prostatectomy, partial and total penectomy, superficial inguinal lymph node dissection, surgery for local tumor recurrence, reconstruction of the urinary tract during surgery for rectal tumors, and excision of pelvic sarcomas.

Dr. James Montie, a close associate, contributed one of the sections on continent urinary diversion. He has developed a new procedure utilizing absorbable staples. Dr. Eti Gursel developed the chapter on myocutaneous flaps in conjunction with the author.

The atlas contains 50 plates that are notable for their wealth of anatomic detail and adherence to surgical perspective. They were drawn by the distinguished medical artist William Loechel. In an era of computer-generated images, he has preserved the craftmanship and skills necessary to render realistic anatomic drawings with superb clarity and fidelity.

J. Edson Pontes, M.D.

Chapter 1

Anatomy of the Pelvis

A large number of the genitourinary organs commonly approached by urologists are located in the pelvis. The pelvic cavity is the lower extension of the abdominal cavity [Hollinshead, 1956]. The "false" pelvis is bounded laterally by the iliac wings, while the "true" pelvis is surrounded posteriorly by the sacrum and anteriorly by the lower portion of the innominate bones, including the pubic rami. The importance of anatomic knowledge of the pelvic cavity and boundaries to the urological surgeon lies in the fact that the relationship of the urinary organs to the bony pelvis will aid in the recognition of genitourinary pathology and in the planning of surgical approaches.

I will describe the important features of the bony pelvis, ligaments, muscles, vessels and nerves, and the organs located in the pelvis.

The Bony Pelvis

The bony pelvis forms a ring which contains the abdominal contents; these are bounded at the lower end by the pelvic floor formed by muscles and ligaments (Figure 1.1). The bony pelvis is formed by the sacrum and coccyx posteriorly, and by the two innominate bones laterally, the latter curving anteriorly to form the pubic rami, which meet each other at the symphysis (Figure 1.1).

Highlights of anatomical landmarks that are often used to plan a surgical approach or are used during surgery are illustrated in Figure 1.1: the anterosuperior iliac spine, which is often used as a landmark to make incisions for approaching the lower ureter; the sacrum promontory, used as a guide to bring the left ureter under the sigmoid during urinary diversion; the obturator foramen, by which the obturator nerve leaves the pelvis; the pubic rami, which must be resected in the rare cases when pubectomy is needed during pelvic surgery. A posterior and lateral view of the bony pelvis is illustrated in Figures 1.2 and 1.3. Although they are of less importance to a urologist, the anatomic landmarks shown in these figures are often used to define the areas of resection needed during combined cases with orthopedic surgeons for large pelvic sarcomas (Chapter 8).

Figure 1.1   *The bony pelvis. Superior anterior view.*

Figure 1.2   *The bony pelvis. Posterior view.*

Figure 1.3   *The bony pelvis. Lateral view.*

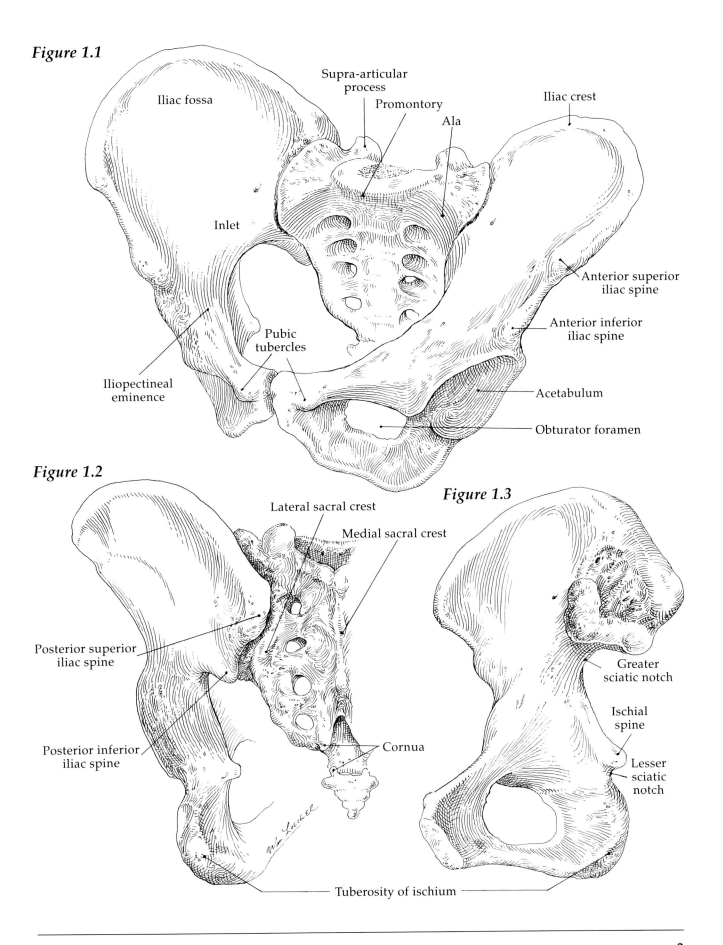

Figure 1.1

Iliac fossa

Supra-articular process

Promontory

Ala

Iliac crest

Inlet

Pubic tubercles

Iliopectineal eminence

Anterior superior iliac spine

Anterior inferior iliac spine

Acetabulum

Obturator foramen

Figure 1.2

Lateral sacral crest

Medial sacral crest

Figure 1.3

Posterior superior iliac spine

Posterior inferior iliac spine

Cornua

Greater sciatic notch

Ischial spine

Lesser sciatic notch

Tuberosity of ischium

The Bony Pelvis

3

Muscles and Ligaments

The ligaments of the pelvis shown in Figures 1.4 to 1.6 are of less importance to the urologic surgeon than the landmarks of the bony pelvis, since they are rarely encountered during surgical procedures, with the exception of the ligaments of the pubic rami and the inguinal ligament. The latter is an important landmark during superficial lymph node dissection for penile cancer (Chapter 6). In this context, the attachment of the sartorius muscle near the anterior iliac spine is of importance because its detachment is necessary to cover the femoral vessels during superficial inguinal node dissection by its reinsertion at the inguinal ligament (Chapter 6).

The muscles lining the pelvis are not often encountered during urologic surgery, with the exception of the psoas muscle (Figure 1.7), which is often used as a landmark posteriorly, and as an anchor during a psoas hitch operation (Chapter 2). The muscles and fascia of the pelvic floor are of great importance to the urologist, since they are in an area frequently encountered during prostatic and bladder surgery (Figures 1.7 to 1.9). A lateral view of the pelvic outlet is shown in Figure 1.10, with identification of the muscles which make up the pelvic floor. The deep and superficial transverse perineal muscles form the urogenital diaphragm (Figures 1.11 and 1.12). Other important areas shown in the view are the puboprostatic ligaments and the rectourethralis muscle, both of which are seen during radical prostatectomy (Figure 1.11).

The levator ani has been described as one of the most variable muscles in the human body [Hollinshead, 1956]. The line of origin of the levator ani from the obturator fascia is called the tendinous arch or white line (Figure 1.10). The levator ani has several components, and is often described as having three main branches: the iliococcygeus, pubococcygeus, and puborectalis muscle (Figures 1.10 and 1.11). The levator ani and its several components form the main part of the pelvic diaphragm [Hollinshead, 1956].

Figure 1.4   *Ligaments of the pelvis. Superior anterior view.*

Figure 1.5   *Ligaments of the pelvis. Posterior view.*

Figure 1.6   *Ligaments of the pelvis. Lateral view.*

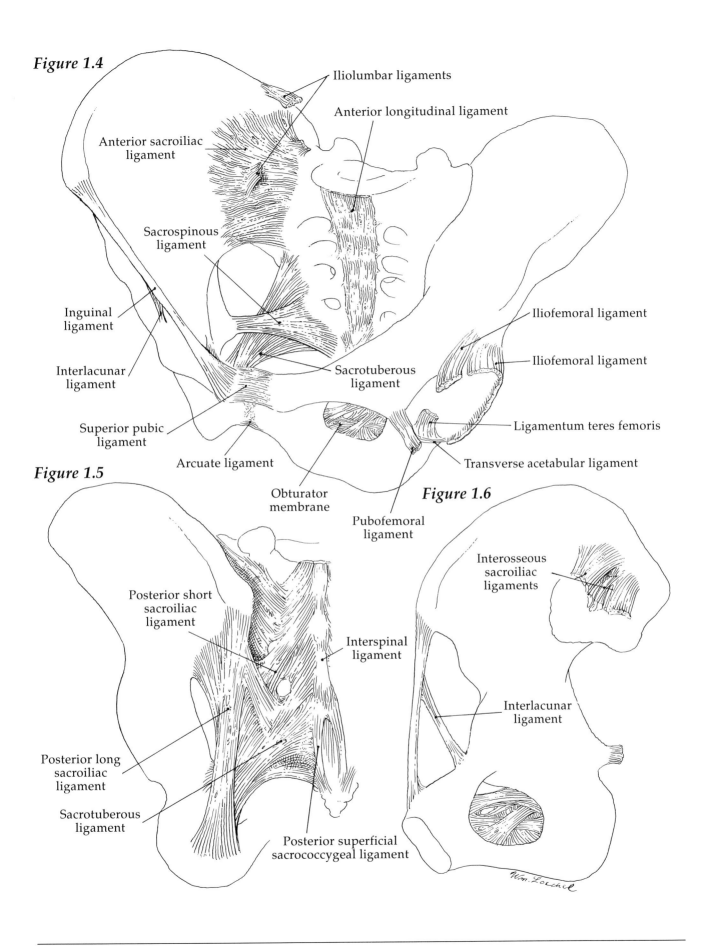

Figure 1.4

Iliolumbar ligaments

Anterior longitudinal ligament

Anterior sacroiliac ligament

Sacrospinous ligament

Inguinal ligament

Interlacunar ligament

Superior pubic ligament

Arcuate ligament

Obturator membrane

Sacrotuberous ligament

Iliofemoral ligament

Iliofemoral ligament

Ligamentum teres femoris

Transverse acetabular ligament

Pubofemoral ligament

Figure 1.5

Posterior short sacroiliac ligament

Interspinal ligament

Posterior long sacroiliac ligament

Sacrotuberous ligament

Posterior superficial sacrococcygeal ligament

Figure 1.6

Interosseous sacroiliac ligaments

Interlacunar ligament

Muscles and Ligaments

5

Figure 1.7   *Muscles of the pelvis. Superior anterior view.*

Figure 1.8   *Muscles of the pelvis. Posterior view.*

Figure 1.9   *Muscles of the pelvis. Lateral view.*

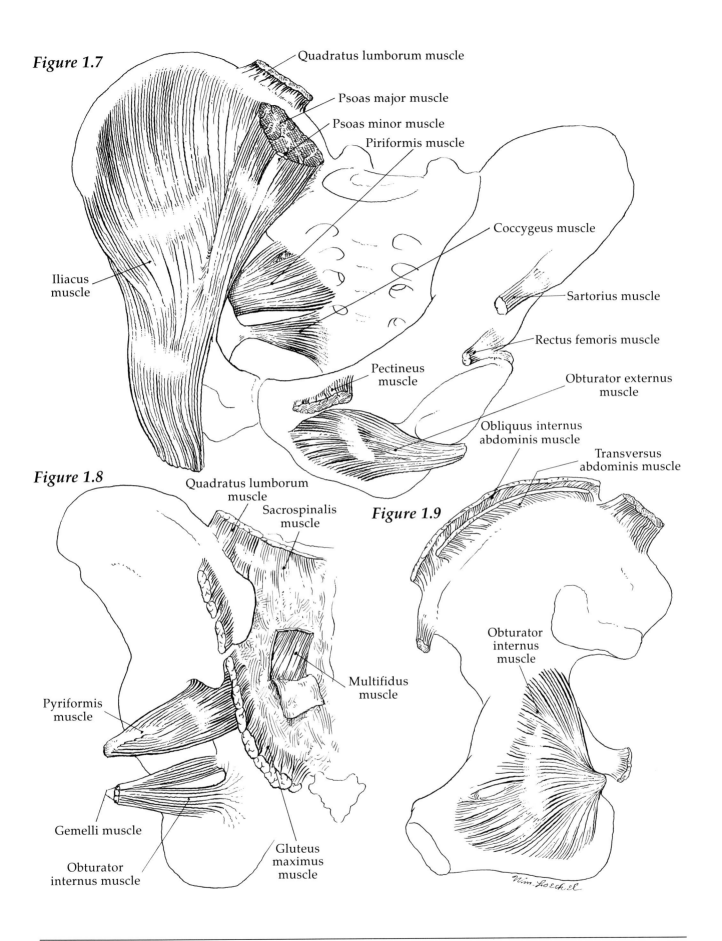

Figure 1.7

Quadratus lumborum muscle

Psoas major muscle

Psoas minor muscle

Piriformis muscle

Coccygeus muscle

Iliacus muscle

Sartorius muscle

Rectus femoris muscle

Pectineus muscle

Obturator externus muscle

Obliquus internus abdominis muscle

Transversus abdominis muscle

Figure 1.8

Quadratus lumborum muscle

Sacrospinalis muscle

Figure 1.9

Obturator internus muscle

Multifidus muscle

Pyriformis muscle

Gemelli muscle

Obturator internus muscle

Gluteus maximus muscle

Figure 1.10 The pelvic outlet. Lateral view. Muscles of the pelvic floor.

Figure 1.11 Urogenital diaphragm. Deep transverse perineal muscles.

Figure 1.12 Urogenital diaphragm. Superficial transverse perineal muscles.

Muscles and Ligaments

Figure 1.10

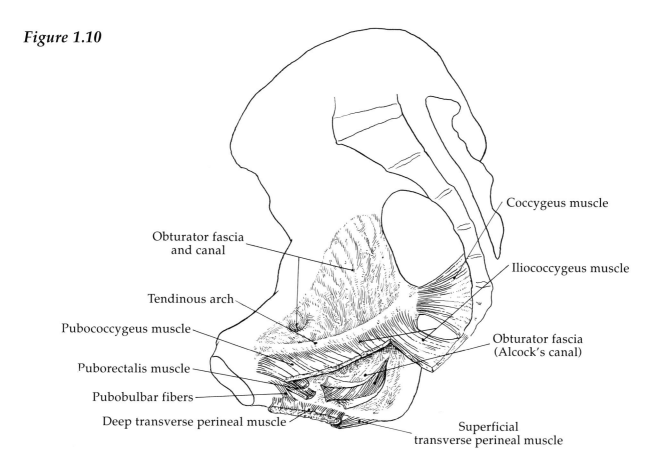

Coccygeus muscle

Obturator fascia
and canal

Iliococcygeus muscle

Tendinous arch

Pubococcygeus muscle

Obturator fascia
(Alcock's canal)

Puborectalis muscle

Pubobulbar fibers

Deep transverse perineal muscle

Superficial
transverse perineal muscle

Figure 1.11

Sacrotuberous ligament

Figure 1.12

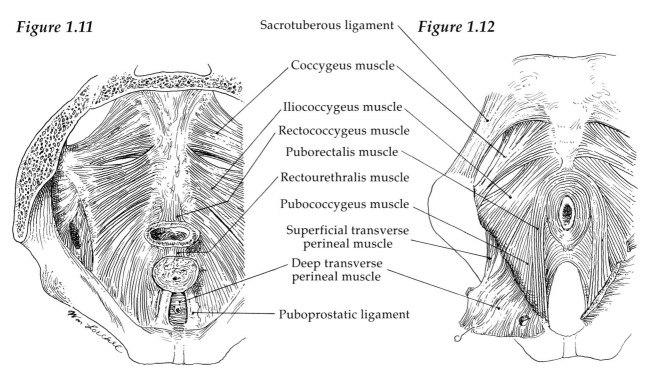

Coccygeus muscle

Iliococcygeus muscle

Rectococcygeus muscle

Puborectalis muscle

Rectourethralis muscle

Pubococcygeus muscle

Superficial transverse
perineal muscle

Deep transverse
perineal muscle

Puboprostatic ligament

Nerves and Plexuses

The nerves and plexuses of the pelvis lie in the lateral pelvic wall, with individual branches to viscera traveling along the fascial planes of these organs [Hollinshead, 1956]. Shown in Figures 1.13 and 1.14 are the origin of the sacral plexus and its muscular relationships. Most of the nerves, as they exit their foramina, are covered by the musculature of the pelvis. Of interest to the urological surgeon are the obturator nerve, which needs to be identified and preserved during pelvic lymph node dissection; the genitofemoral nerve, used as a landmark during pelvic lymphadenectomy; and the femoral nerve, which needs to be identified during superficial inguinal node dissection, and which occasionally may be submitted to stretch injury during surgery for pelvic malignancy [Hollinshead, 1956].

The Autonomic Nervous System

The anatomy of the hypogastric plexus is highly complicated because of its many extensions, both its subdivisions which join the splenic fibers of the sacral nerves and its parasympathetic fibers to the viscera (Figure 1.15) [Gardner, 1975]. Of particular importance are the prostatic plexus, which can be identified and kept intact in the course of radical prostatectomy in order to preserve erectile function (Chapter 5). Because of its extensive network and connections, branches of the autonomic nervous system may be damaged during pelvic surgery such as abdominal perineal resection for rectal cancer. Such damage may result in bladder dysfunction.

Figure 1.13   Origin of the sacral plexus. Superior anterior view.

Figure 1.14   Origin of the sacral plexus. Lateral view.

Figure 1.15   Hypogastric plexus. Lateral view.

Figure 1.13

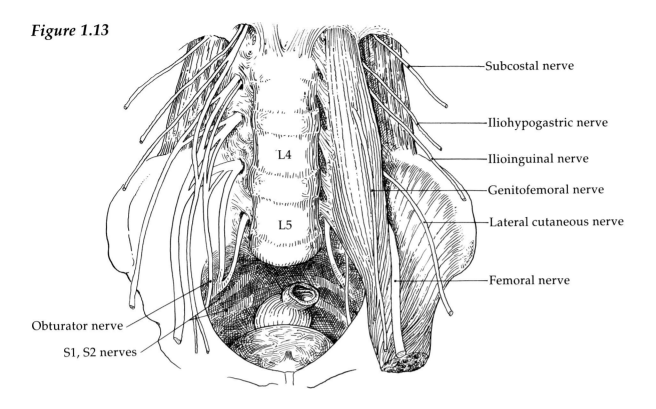

Subcostal nerve

Iliohypogastric nerve

Ilioinguinal nerve

Genitofemoral nerve

Lateral cutaneous nerve

Femoral nerve

L4

L5

Obturator nerve

S1, S2 nerves

Figure 1.14

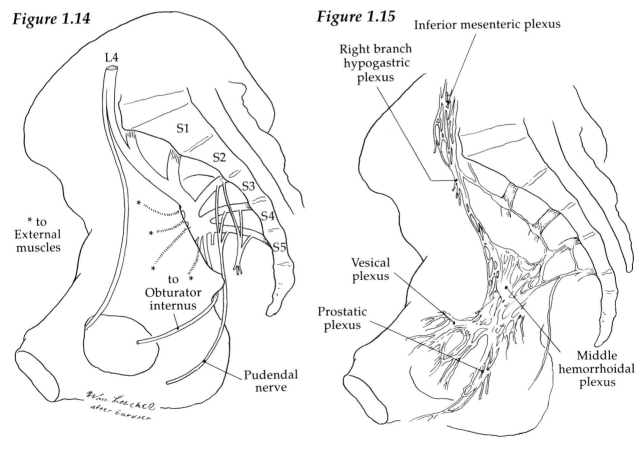

L4

S1

S2

S3

S4

S5

* to
External
muscles

to
Obturator
internus

Pudendal
nerve

Wm. Loechel
after Gardner

Figure 1.15

Inferior mesenteric plexus

Right branch
hypogastric
plexus

Vesical
plexus

Prostatic
plexus

Middle
hemorrhoidal
plexus

Nerves and Plexuses and The Autonomic Nervous System

11

The Vascular System

The arterial and venous system of the pelvis is shown in Figure 1.16. The common iliac artery divides into the external iliac artery and the internal iliac, or hypogastric, artery. The external iliac artery never enters the true pelvis. It lies laterally over the muscles covering the innominate bone and exits at the femoral ring as the femoral artery. The internal iliac artery provides all the arterial branches for vessels in the pelvis, with the exception of the middle sacral and superior rectal (hemorrhoidal) vessels [Hollinshead, 1956].

The obturator vessels coursing around the obturator nerve, and the relationship of the ureter and the uterine artery, are shown in Figure 1.17. The internal iliac artery arises from the common iliac artery at the level of the lumbosacral articulation and, as it enters the true pelvis, is separated from the psoas muscle by the external iliac vein. Although traditionally two main trunks (anterior and posterior) have been described (the anterior having branches to the viscera of the pelvis, and the posterior to the body wall and buttocks), there are significant anatomical variations. Described in Figure 1.18 is the most common arrangement of those divisions. Note that the superior vesical artery, the first arterial branch of the hypogastric artery, is ligated initially during the course of cystectomy.

Figure 1.16   *Arterial and venous system of the pelvis.*

Figure 1.17   *Relationship of the ureter and uterine artery.*

Figure 1.18   *Iliac arteries—common, internal, and external. Lateral view.*

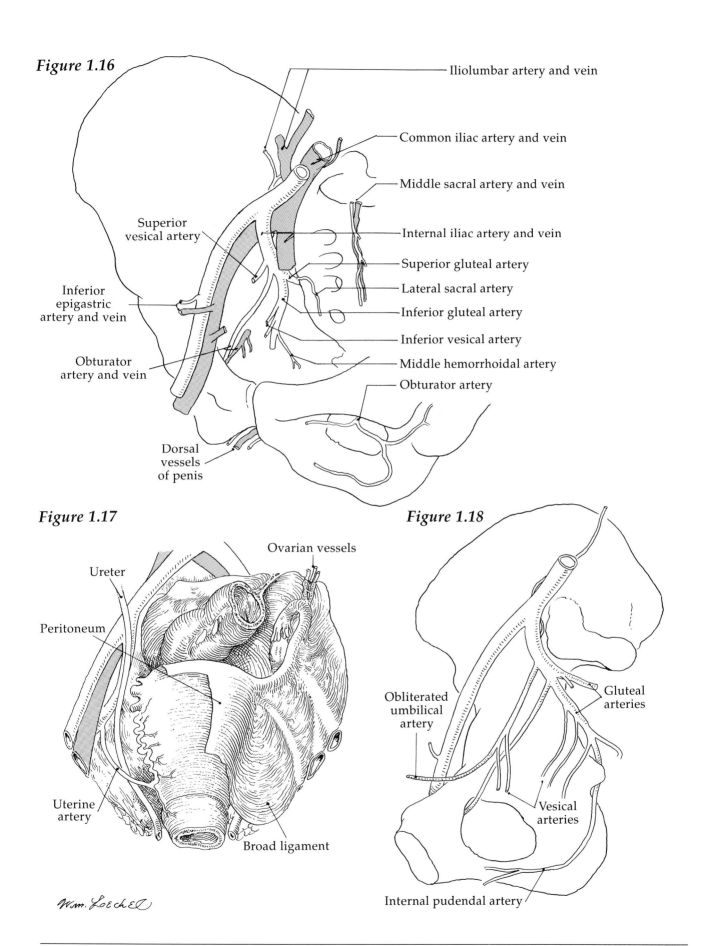

Figure 1.16

Iliolumbar artery and vein

Common iliac artery and vein

Middle sacral artery and vein

Superior vesical artery

Internal iliac artery and vein

Superior gluteal artery

Lateral sacral artery

Inferior gluteal artery

Inferior epigastric artery and vein

Inferior vesical artery

Middle hemorrhoidal artery

Obturator artery and vein

Obturator artery

Dorsal vessels of penis

Figure 1.17

Ureter

Ovarian vessels

Peritoneum

Uterine artery

Broad ligament

Wm. Loechel

Figure 1.18

Obliterated umbilical artery

Gluteal arteries

Vesical arteries

Internal pudendal artery

The Vascular System

13

Urogenital Organs in the Pelvis

The Pelvic Ureter

The pelvic portion of the ureter follows a similar course in men and women. The relationships of the lower ureter in the deep pelvis are somewhat different because of the different organs and structures encountered in the different sexual organs. After crossing the pelvic brim at the level of the bifurcation of the iliac artery, the ureter runs downwards until it medially enters the tissue of the sacral-genital fold and the urinary bladder. Each ureter passes medially to the obturator nerve and vessels. In men, the ureter is crossed on its medial side by the vas deferens, which courses posteriorly to the ureter before converging medially to enter the prostate. In women, in the upper part of its course, it lies posterior to the ovaries [Hollinshead, 1956]. As the ureter moves downward it enters the lateral cervical ligament at the base of the broad ligament passing behind the uterine artery, and then enters the bladder (Figure 1.17) [Hollinshead, 1956].

The Urinary Bladder

In the adult, the bladder lies deep in the pelvis behind the pubic rami and, depending on the degree of fullness, it contacts the anterior abdominal wall. The neck of the bladder in a male is in intimate contact with the prostate, which surrounds the proximal part of the urethra. In the female, the neck of the bladder is in direct contact with the pubococcygeus portion of the levator ani [Hollinshead, 1956]. Posterior to the bladder in a male are the seminal vesicles and in the female the vagina (Figures 1.19 and 1.20). The relationships of the bladder to its surrounding organs are illustrated for the male and female in Figures 1.19 and 1.20.

Figure 1.19 Urinary bladder and surrounding structures. Male.

Figure 1.20 Urinary bladder and surrounding structures. Female.

Figure 1.19

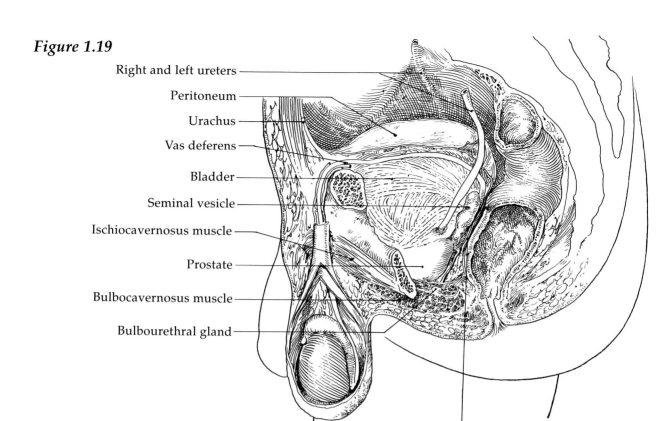

Right and left ureters

Peritoneum

Urachus

Vas deferens

Bladder

Seminal vesicle

Ischiocavernosus muscle

Prostate

Bulbocavernosus muscle

Bulbourethral gland

Rectovesical septum
(Denonvilliers' fascia)

Figure 1.20

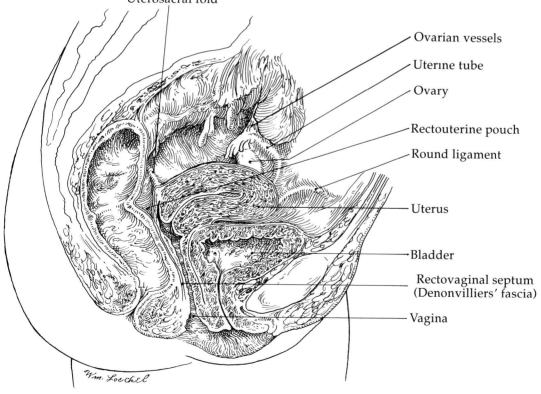

Uterosacral fold

Ovarian vessels

Uterine tube

Ovary

Rectouterine pouch

Round ligament

Uterus

Bladder

Rectovaginal septum
(Denonvilliers' fascia)

Vagina

Wm. Loechel

Urogenital Organs in the Pelvis

The Prostate

The prostate gland surrounds the urethra as it exits the bladder. Therefore, at its base it is in close contact with the bladder neck, and at its apex it rests against the upper surface of the levator ani. Covering the prostate on its lateral and apical aspect is the endopelvic fascia, which needs to be open at the initiation of radical prostatectomy for complete mobilization of the prostate (Chapter 5). The fibers of the pubococcygeus muscle on both sides of the prostate are in close contact with the gland and have, for this reason, been called the levator prostate. These fibers must be isolated and divided from the prostate during radical prostatectomy, as they are a significant source of bleeding during that operation (Chapter 5). Anteriorly, the prostate is attached to the pubis by the puboprostatic ligaments, which need to be divided during radical prostatectomy (Chapter 5). Between the puboprostatic ligaments, overlying the urethra and apex of the prostate, lies the dorsal vein of the penis complex which needs to be controlled at the time of radical prostatectomy (Chapter 5). The prostate is surrounded anteriorly and laterally by a considerable quantity of connective tissue. Posteriorly, the prostatoperitoneal membrane or rectovesical septum (Denonvilliers' fascia) separates the prostate from the rectum, and extends up and around the seminal vesicles (Figure 1.19). In women, the same fascia exists and is located behind the vagina (Figure 1.20).

Chapter 2

Surgery of the Bladder and Lower Ureter

Partial Cystectomy

Indications for partial cystectomy in invasive bladder cancer include unifocal tumors located in the anterior or dome of the bladder, which can be resected with a tumor-free margin and preservation of a functional organ. Only about 5% of all patients seen are ideal candidates for this procedure [Pontes, 1991]. A midline vertical intraperitoneal incision is performed (Figure 2.1). After a bilateral lymph node dissection (Figures 2.14 to 2.17), the bladder is dissected carefully. The area of the tumor is palpated gently to allow delineation of the area of normal bladder to be excised. The peritoneal covering of the bladder is included in the resection (Figures 2.2 and 2.3). Careful packing to avoid tumor spillage is important. The tumor and a 2-cm margin of normal bladder is excised. At the edges of the remaining bladder wound four-quadrant biopsies are done to ascertain negative margins (Figures 2.4 and 2.5). The bladder is closed in two layers (Figure 2.6). A Foley catheter is left in the urethra for seven to ten days. Closed system drains are left in both sides of the node dissection.

Figure 2.1   *Partial cystectomy. Midline vertical intraperitoneal incision for removing tumor of the anterior bladder (inset).*

Figure 2.2   *Partial cystectomy. Dissection of the bladder, with packing to avoid tumor spillage.*

Figure 2.3   *Partial cystectomy. Palpation of the tumor and delineation of the area of excision.*

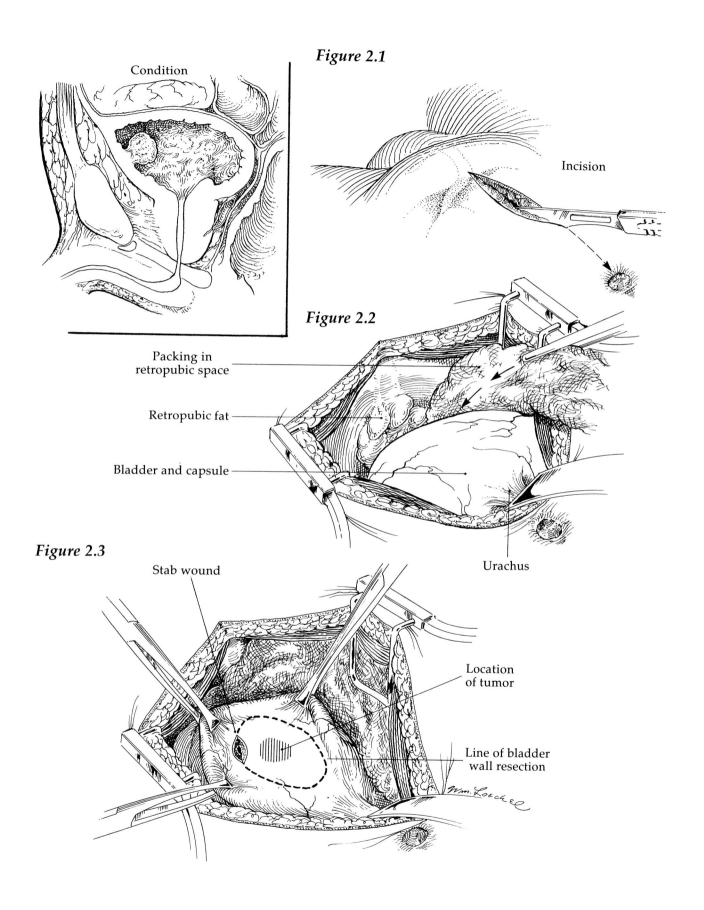

Figure 2.1

Condition

Incision

Figure 2.2

Packing in
retropubic space

Retropubic fat

Bladder and capsule

Urachus

Figure 2.3

Stab wound

Location
of tumor

Line of bladder
wall resection

Figure 2.4 *Partial cystectomy. Excision of the tumor with a 2-cm margin of normal bladder.*

Figure 2.5 *Partial cystectomy. Four-quadrant biopsy at the edges of the bladder wound.*

Figure 2.6 *Partial cystectomy. Closure of the bladder in two layers.*

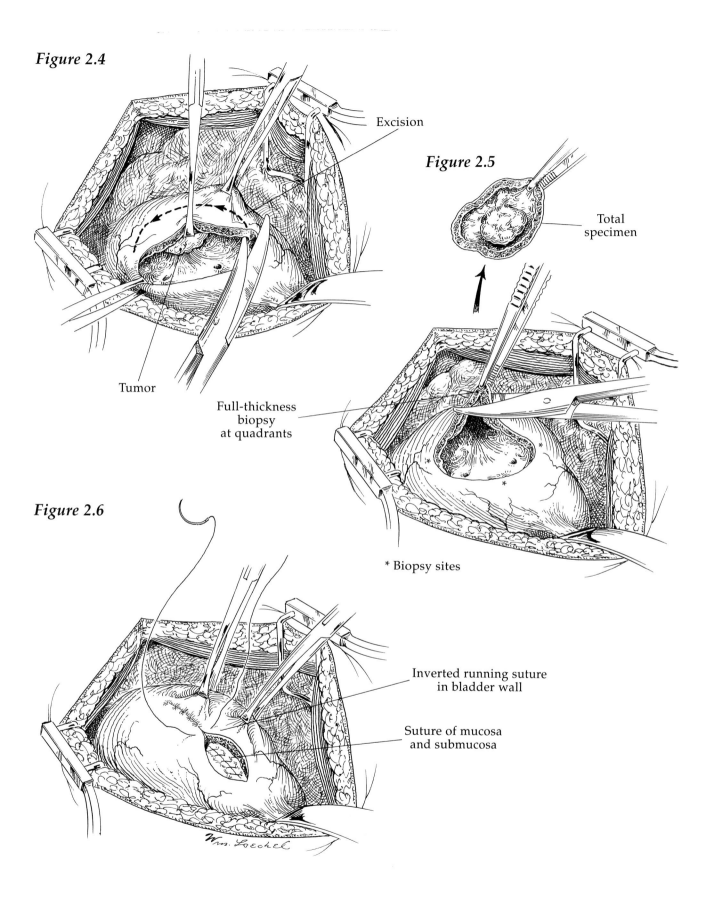

Figure 2.4

Excision

Figure 2.5

Total
specimen

Tumor

Full-thickness
biopsy
at quadrants

* Biopsy sites

Figure 2.6

Inverted running suture
in bladder wall

Suture of mucosa
and submucosa

Partial Cystectomy

Tumor in a Diverticulum

Bladder diverticulectomy for tumor follows the same principles outlined previously (Figure 2.7). Because bladder diverticula are usually laterally or posterolaterally located, identification and isolation of the ipsilateral ureter is important (Figure 2.8). The diverticulum with an edge of normal bladder is excised (Figure 2.8 inset). Biopsy of the bladder edges is done to assure negative margins. The bladder is closed in two layers (Figure 2.9). If necessary, reimplantation of the ureter can be done.

Figure 2.7   *Bladder diverticulectomy. Midline vertical intraperitoneal incision for removing a tumor in a diverticulum (inset).*

Figure 2.8   *Bladder diverticulectomy. Isolation of the ipsilateral ureter and excision of the diverticulum.*

Figure 2.9   *Bladder diverticulectomy. Closure of the bladder in two layers.*

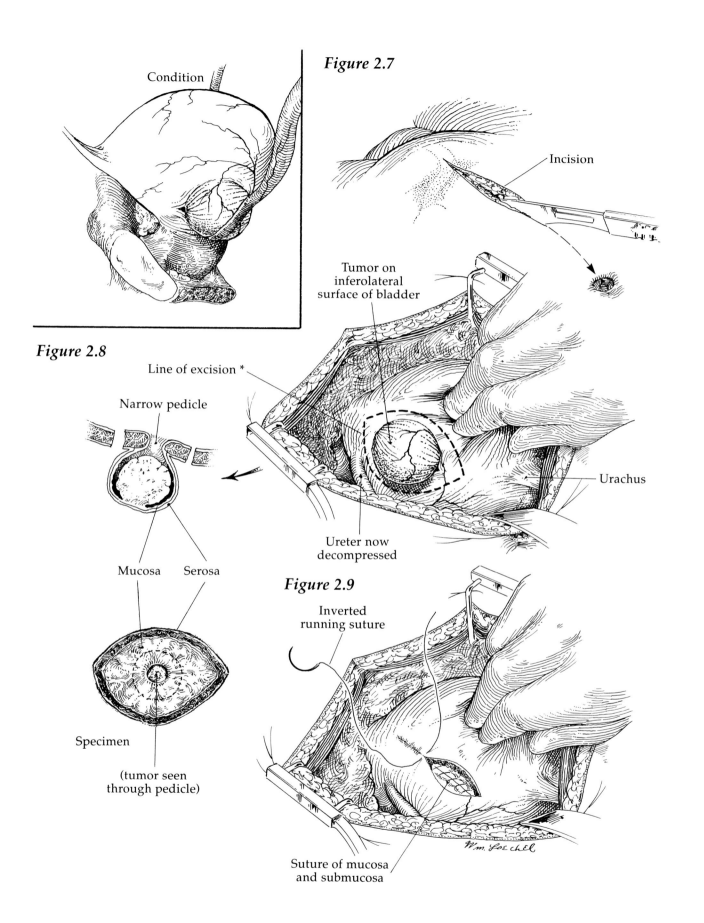

Condition

Figure 2.7

Incision

Tumor on
inferolateral
surface of bladder

Urachus

Line of excision *

Ureter now
decompressed

Figure 2.8

Narrow pedicle

Mucosa   Serosa

Specimen

(tumor seen
through pedicle)

Figure 2.9

Inverted
running suture

Suture of mucosa
and submucosa

Partial Cystectomy for Tumors Located Near the Ureteral Orifice

Illustrated in the inset is a tumor located at the level of the ureteral orifice. A midline lower abdominal incision is performed (Figure 2.10). The bladder is dissected, isolating the ureter on the affected side; it is opened, taking the same precautions to avoid tumor spillage as in partial cystectomy. The tumor is excised with the wide margin of normal bladder including the distal ureter (Figure 2.11). The tumor and distal ureter are removed (Figure 2.12), and the bladder is closed in two layers as shown previously (Figure 2.9).

Figures 2.10 and 2.11 *Partial cystectomy for a tumor near the ureteral orifice.*

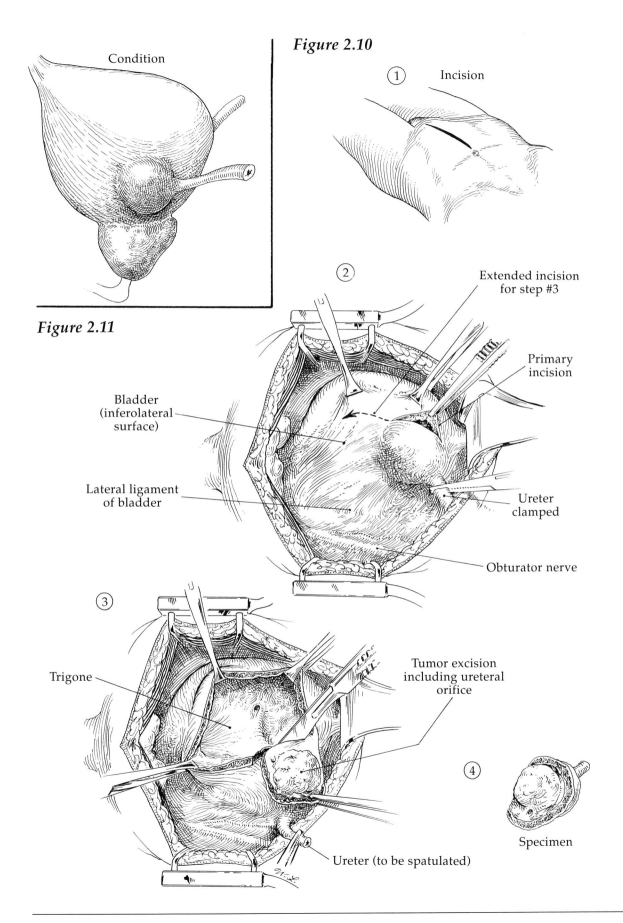

Condition

Figure 2.10

① Incision

Figure 2.11

② Extended incision for step #3

Primary incision

Bladder (inferolateral surface)

Lateral ligament of bladder

Ureter clamped

Obturator nerve

③ Trigone

Tumor excision including ureteral orifice

④ Specimen

Ureter (to be spatulated)

Distal Ureterectomy–
Ureteral Reimplant

Ureteral reimplant needs to be done either as part of an excision of a lower ureteral tumor or as part of a partial cystectomy which involves the ureteral orifice. The simplest modality of ureteral reimplant is a direct anastomosis (fish-mouth) in the dome of the bladder (Figure 2.12). In the normal ureter, spatulation of the lumen is necessary to prevent obstruction. When the ureteral lumen is anastomosed to the bladder, mucosa (4-0 polyglycol) fixation of the ureter to the serosa is recommended to relieve tension. Adults tolerate this type of reimplant reasonably well although it is associated with vesicoureteral reflux. When a larger segment of the ureter is resected, a psoas hitch, in which the bladder wall is sutured to the psoas on the ipsilateral side, will bridge the gap (Figure 2.13).

Figure 2.12 Distal ureterectomy. Ureteral implant; direct anastomosis (fish-mouth) in the dome of the bladder.

Figure 2.13 Distal ureterectomy. Ureteral implant; psoas hitch. The bladder wall is sutured to the psoas on the ipsilateral side.

Figure 2.12

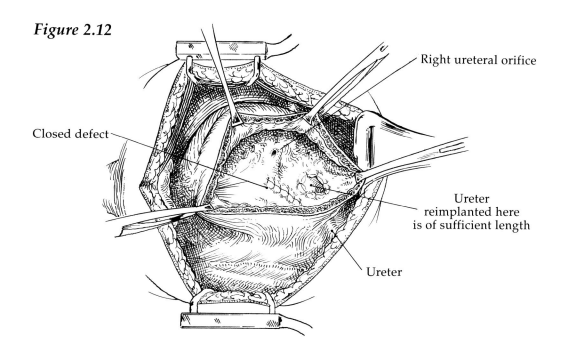

Right ureteral orifice

Closed defect

Ureter
reimplanted here
is of sufficient length

Ureter

Figure 2.13

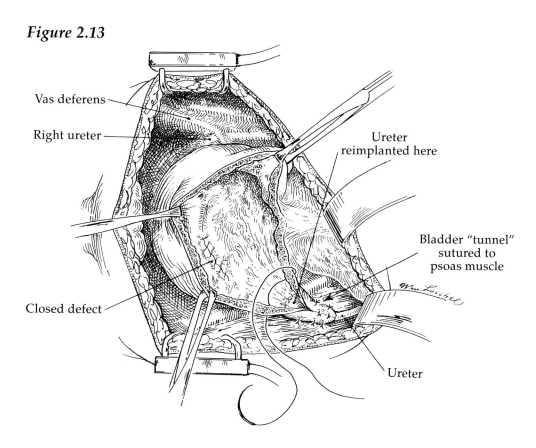

Vas deferens

Right ureter

Ureter
reimplanted here

Bladder "tunnel"
sutured to
psoas muscle

Closed defect

Ureter

Pelvic Lymphadenectomy

Pelvic lymphadenectomy is now a standard procedure in the surgical excision of malignant neoplasms. Controversy exists regarding its effectiveness as curative procedure versus its use for a staging, i.e., defining the extent of disease and evaluating prognostic factors.

Because most surgeons now accept the value of lymphadenectomy as a staging rather than a curative procedure, modified lymphadenectomy, which provides information regarding the status of the primary involved nodes, and at the same time decreases morbidity, is being used especially in association with radical prostatectomy.

Pelvic Lymphadenectomy in Bladder Cancer

A midline transabdominal incision is performed (Figure 2.14). After the placement of a self-retained retractor (Bookwalter), retraction of the small bowel upwards will expose the posterior peritoneum. The common iliac artery is identified on the right side, the posterior peritoneum is incised, and the right ureter isolated and retracted. All the areolar tissues within the limits illustrated are dissected (Figures 2.15 to 2.17). After completion of the procedure, the obturator nerve is clearly identified and preserved. On the left side, the sigmoid colon has to be retracted medially to expose the vessels as on the right side. The limits of dissection have been indicated previously (Figure 2.17).

Figure 2.14   *Pelvic lymphadenectomy. Midline transabdominal incision.*

Figure 2.15   *Pelvic lymphadenectomy. Placement of self-retained retractor (Bookwalter) and retraction of the small bowel upwards to expose the posterior peritoneum.*

Figure 2.16   *Pelvic lymphadenectomy. Identification of the common ileal artery, incision of posterior peritoneum, and isolation and retraction of the right ureter.*

Figure 2.17   *Pelvic lymphadenectomy. Areolar tissues to be dissected.*

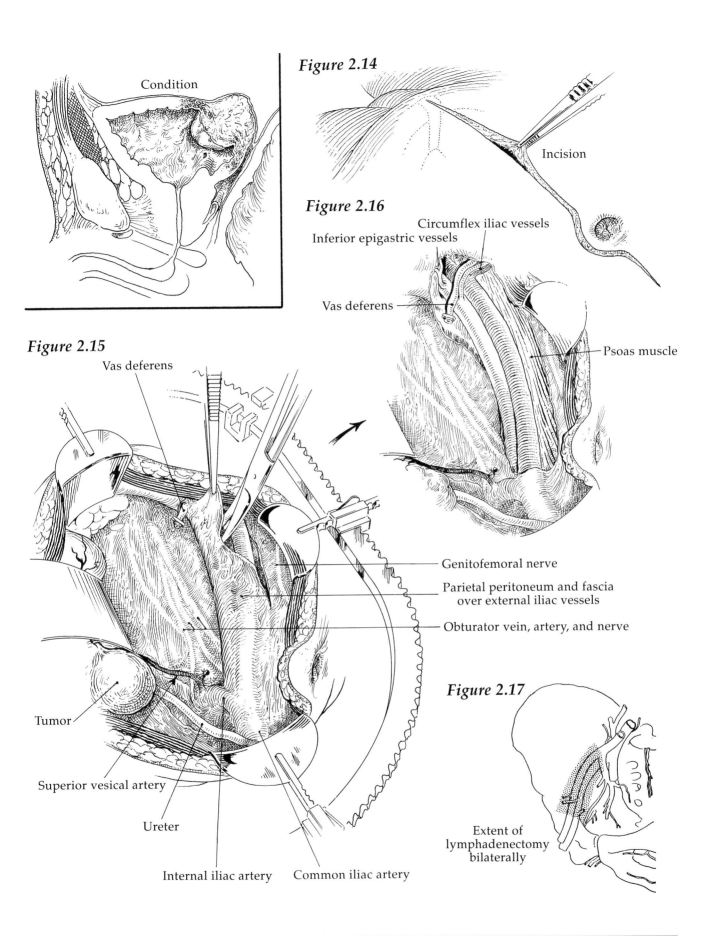

Condition

Figure 2.14

Incision

Figure 2.16

Circumflex iliac vessels

Inferior epigastric vessels

Vas deferens

Psoas muscle

Figure 2.15

Vas deferens

Genitofemoral nerve

Parietal peritoneum and fascia
over external iliac vessels

Obturator vein, artery, and nerve

Tumor

Superior vesical artery

Ureter

Internal iliac artery

Common iliac artery

Figure 2.17

Extent of
lymphadenectomy
bilaterally

Radical Cystectomy

The procedure illustrated here is a variation of the one previously described [Montie, 1983]. The same incision is used as for pelvic lymphadenectomy for bladder cancer. A self-retained retractor is used for exposure of the bladder (Figure 2.18). On each side of the bladder, the vas deferens, the superior vesical artery, and the ureter are ligated and transected (Figure 2.19). Frozen sections of the distal ureter are obtained to assure negative margins. The posterior peritoneum between the bladder and rectum is incised, and by blunt dissection, the bladder is separated from the rectum (Figure 2.20). After this dissection, the bladder pedicles are separated behind the stump of the ureter into the lateral and lateroposterior pedicles. Ligation of the pedicles is done by metal clips, with transection of the tissues between the rows of clips (Figure 2.21). This dissection is done laterally and posteriorly to the level of the base of the prostate. At this point, the procedure is done in a retrograde fashion, like a radical prostatectomy (Figures 2.22 to 2.24 inset). This is particularly important in cases where the urethra needs to be preserved for continent urinary diversion. With this antegrade and retrograde dissection, only small parts of the lateral pedicles remain and these can be ligated with clips. The specimen is removed as illustrated in Figure 2.25. At the end of the procedure, a Foley catheter is left indwelling with a 30-cc balloon to provide hemostasis (Figure 2.26).

Figure 2.18   *Radical cystectomy condition. Midline transabdominal incision. A self-retained retractor exposes the bladder.*

Figure 2.19   *Radical cystectomy. Ligation and transection of the vas deferens and the superior vesical artery.*

Figure 2.20   *Radical cystectomy. Ligation of the ureter and incision of the posterior peritoneum and separation of the bladder from the rectum.*

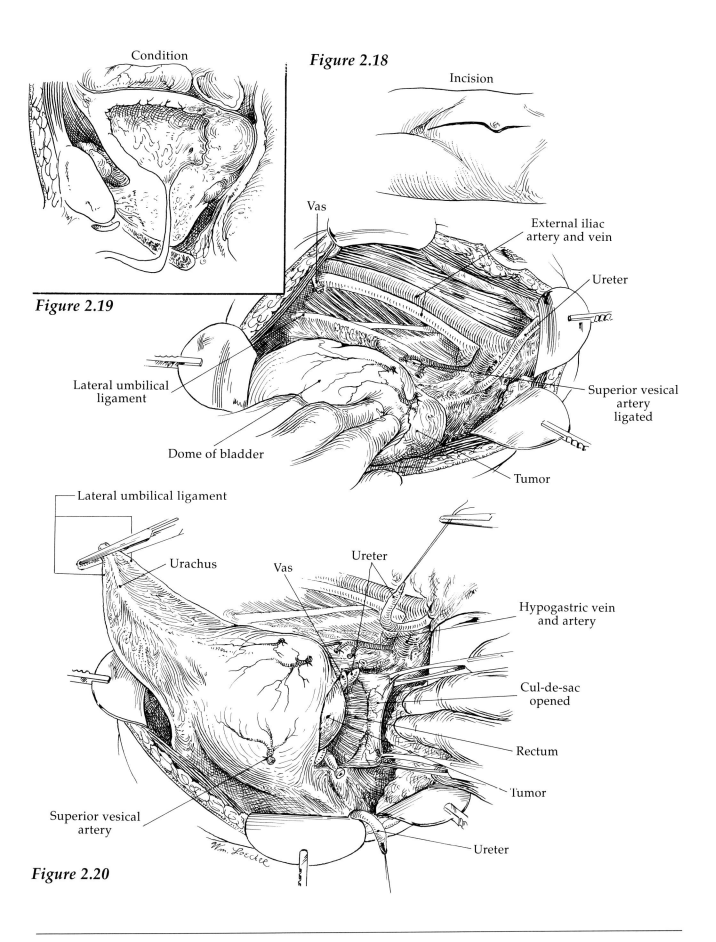

Condition

Figure 2.18

Incision

Figure 2.19

Vas

External iliac
artery and vein

Ureter

Lateral umbilical
ligament

Superior vesical
artery
ligated

Dome of bladder

Tumor

Lateral umbilical ligament

Urachus

Vas

Ureter

Hypogastric vein
and artery

Cul-de-sac
opened

Rectum

Tumor

Superior vesical
artery

Ureter

Figure 2.20

Radical Cystectomy

31

Figure 2.21   *Radical cystectomy. Separation, ligation, and transection of the bladder pedicles.*

Figure 2.22   *Radical cystectomy. Dissection of the pedicles laterally and posteriorly, to the level of the base of the prostate.*

Radical Cystectomy

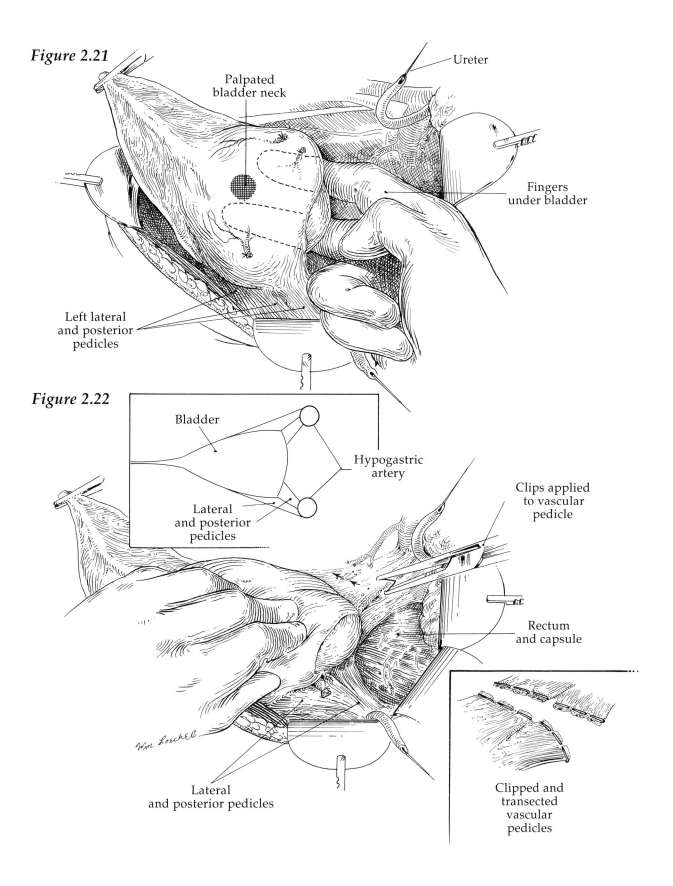

Figure 2.21

Ureter

Palpated
bladder neck

Fingers
under bladder

Left lateral
and posterior
pedicles

Figure 2.22

Bladder

Hypogastric
artery

Lateral
and posterior
pedicles

Clips applied
to vascular
pedicle

Rectum
and capsule

Wm. Loschel

Lateral
and posterior pedicles

Clipped and
transected
vascular
pedicles

Figure 2.23 *Radical cystectomy. Retrograde dissection of the prostate; excision of the puboprostatic ligaments, ligation of the dorsal vein of the penis.*

Figure 2.24 *Radical cystectomy. Incision in the anterior surface of the urethra with exposure of the Foley catheter, which is now used for traction (inset).*

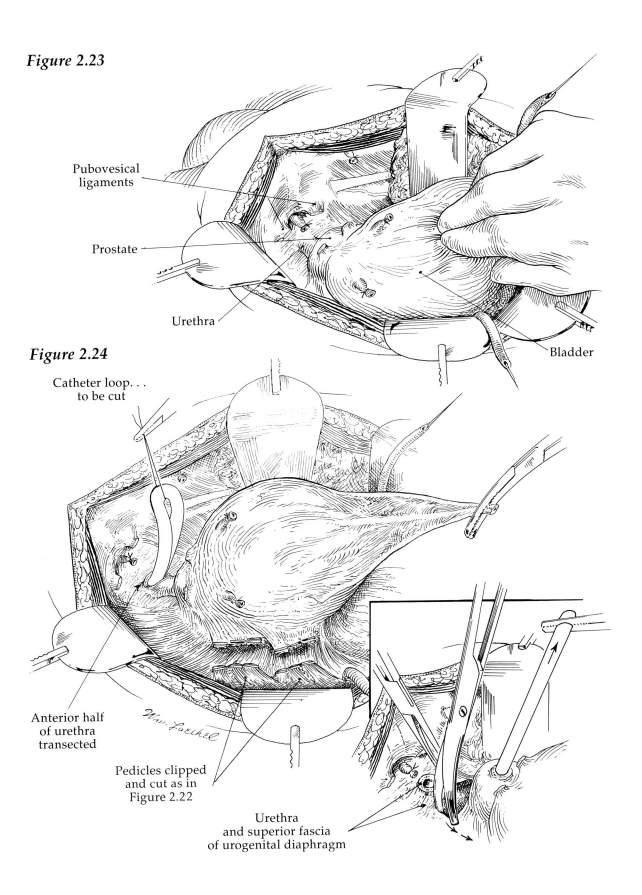

Figure 2.23

Pubovesical
ligaments

Prostate

Urethra

Bladder

Figure 2.24

Catheter loop. . .
to be cut

Anterior half
of urethra
transected

Pedicles clipped
and cut as in
Figure 2.22

Urethra
and superior fascia
of urogenital diaphragm

Figure 2.25   *Radical cystectomy. Excised bladder.*

Figure 2.26   *Radical cystectomy. Indwelling Foley catheter with 30-cc balloon.*

Figure 2.25

Figure 2.26

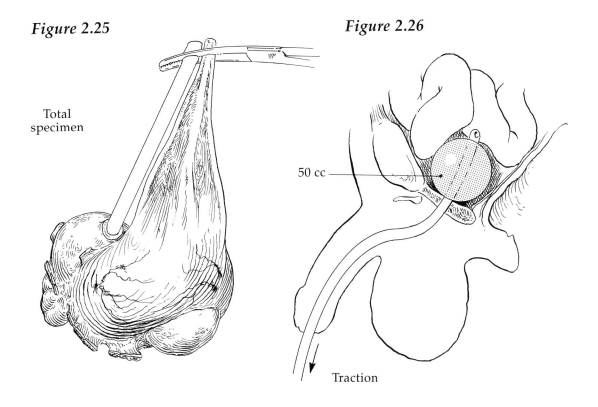

Total
specimen

50 cc

Traction

Radical Cystectomy in Women

The incidence of bladder cancer is significantly lower in women and, therefore, this procedure is not commonly done. The procedure in the female is always an anterior pelvic exenteration. Variation from the cystectomy in males includes positioning of the patient in a modified lithotomy position so as to have access to the urethra which must be included with the specimen, and preparation of the vagina with placement of a roll which can be palpated at the time of surgery. The uterus, fallopian tubes, ovaries, and bladder are removed en bloc with the segment of vagina, the size of which depends on the extent and location of the tumor.

Chapter 3

Urinary Diversion

Urinary diversion following cystectomy can be either diversion with a stoma and the use of an appliance, or continent diversion to the skin or to the urethra. Indications for the different types of urinary diversion have been reviewed recently [Montie et al., 1987].

Noncontinent Urinary Diversion

The most common urinary diversions used are the ileal conduit and ureteroileal anastomosis. For the ileal conduit, a segment of ileum of adequate length, approximately 15 cm from the ileocecal valve, is selected (Figure 3.1). The size of the ileal segment must be individualized to the patient and depends on many factors, e.g., mobility of the mesentery, obesity, and so on. The mesentery is divided to allow mobility of the segment while preserving the vascular supply. This can be done with a cautery knife and ligation of any visible vessels. After a segment of ileum is isolated, reanastomosis of the small bowel is performed using mechanical staples from a GIA and TA-55 device (Figures 3.2 to 3.4).

There are two types of ureteroileal anastomosis, and the choice depends on personal preference or intraoperative circumstances.

Figure 3.1 *Noncontinent urinary diversion. Ileal conduit; ileal segment stapled and immobilized.*

Figure 3.2 *Noncontinent urinary diversion. Ileal conduit; application of linear cutter.*

Figure 3.3 *Noncontinent urinary diversion. Ileal conduit; edges a and b (Figure 3.2) are stapled together.*

Figure 3.4 *Noncontinent urinary diversion. Ileal conduit; anastomosis completed.*

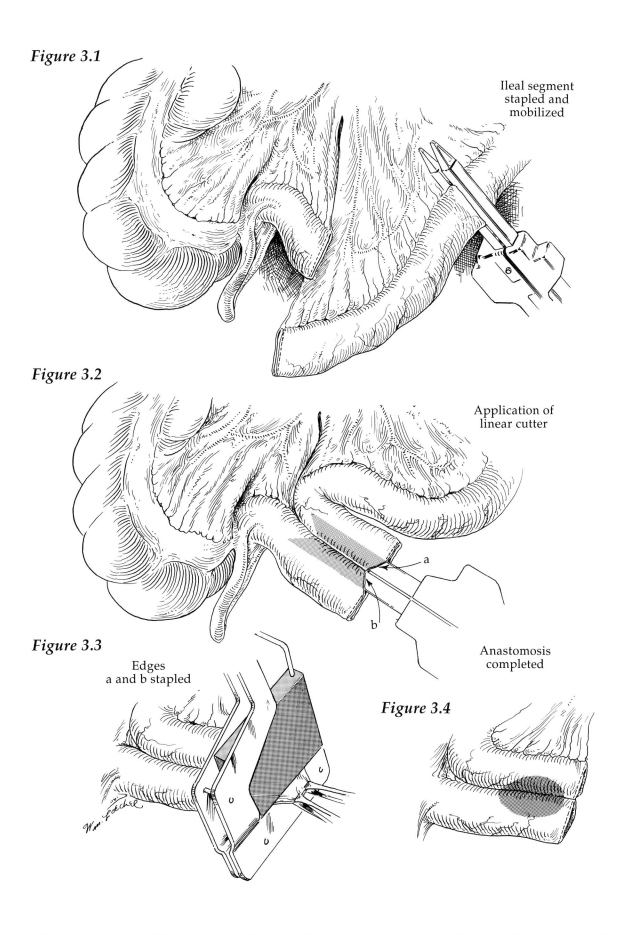

Figure 3.1

Ileal segment
stapled and
mobilized

Figure 3.2

Application of
linear cutter

a

b

Figure 3.3

Edges
a and b stapled

Anastomosis
completed

Figure 3.4

Bricker Ureteroileal Anastomosis

The ureters are mobilized and transected as part of the cystectomy. Stay sutures are placed on the posterior lip of the ureters. The ureters are brought in close proximity to the ileal segment (Figure 3.5).

A site for the anastomosis between the ureters and the ileum is chosen. This site should be 3 to 4 cm from the end of the loop with a distance of 3 to 4 cm between the ureters. The ureters are spatulated anteriorly to a distance of 1.5 to 2 cm. A stay suture of 5-0 polyglycol, which will be used later in the anastomosis, is placed at the apex of the spatulated end. By manipulating the ureter, a site for the ileal incision is chosen near the antimesentery border. A small incision is made in the bowel's serosa and muscularis with protrusion of the mucosa and a small segment of the mucosa is excised. A stay suture of 5-0 polyglycol is placed at the distal edge of this incision to provide exposure during the anastomosis and to be used for the last suture of the ureteroileal anastomosis.

The anastomosis is started by placing a 4-0 silk suture between the serosa of the bowel and the serosa of the ureter to fix the ureter to the bowel and thus prevent tension in the anastomosis. The stay suture placed at the corner of the spatulated ureter is now used to initiate the ureteroileal anastomosis. The anastomosis is done with interrupted 5-0 polyglycol sutures (Figure 3.5). Before completion, a #8 feeding tube is placed upward in the ureter to assure patency. No stents are left indwelling.

Figure 3.5 *Noncontinent urinary diversion. Bricker ureteroileal anastomosis.*

Figure 3.5
Bricker

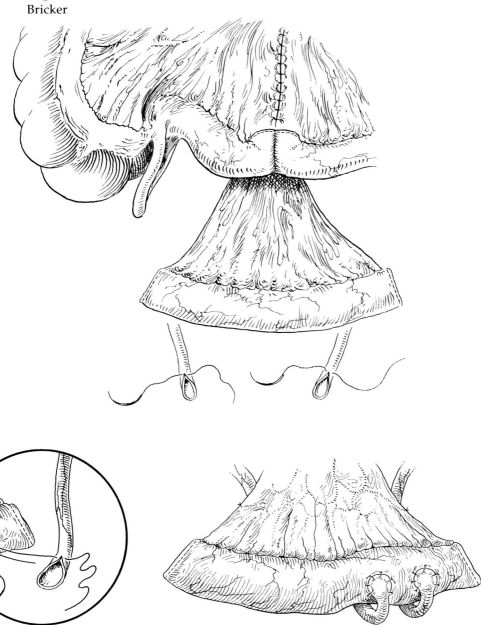

Wallace Ureteroileal Anastomosis

The stapled end of the ileal conduit is removed, leaving that end ready to be used in the anastomosis. The ureters are spatulated on their anterior border to a distance approximating the diameter of the ileal conduit. A side-to-side anastomosis with a running 5-0 polyglycol suture is performed (Figure 3.6 inset). The joined ureters are anastomosed to the end of the ileal conduit (Figure 3.6).

The location of the stoma is chosen the day before surgery by the stoma therapy team. More than one location is selected to provide flexibility at the time of surgery. A skin incision at the chosen location is made with removal of the skin and some of the underlying fat. The fascia of the external oblique muscle is incised and a small segment removed. The underlying muscle fibers are separated, and a small window of the peritoneum is removed. This incision should allow comfortably for two finger-breadths. If the incision is too tight, it may compromise the blood supply of the ileal segment, and if too large, it may lead to parastomal hernia.

In the end stoma (Figure 3.7), the end of the ileal conduit is brought to the skin and everting sutures are used.

In the Turnbull stoma, the end is kept closed, a small opening in the mesenteric part of the bowel is made 2 cm from the end, a half-inch umbilical tape is passed through, and the ileum is brought to the skin as a loop. Once the ileum is at skin level the umbilical tape is removed and replaced by a plastic rod. The antimesenteric portion of the ileum is then incised, and the bowel everted (Figure 3.8).

Figure 3.6 Noncontinent urinary diversion. Wallace ureteroileal anastomosis.

Figure 3.7 Noncontinent urinary diversion. Ileal conduit; end stoma with everting sutures.

Figure 3.8 Noncontinent urinary diversion. Ileal conduit; Turnbull stoma with everted bowel.

Figure 3.6
Wallace

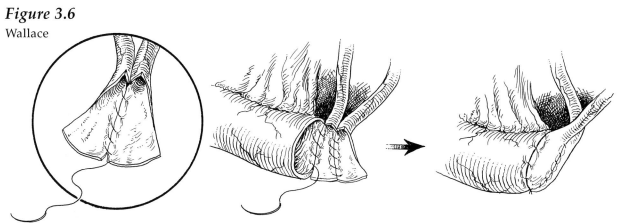

Figure 3.7
End stoma (a)

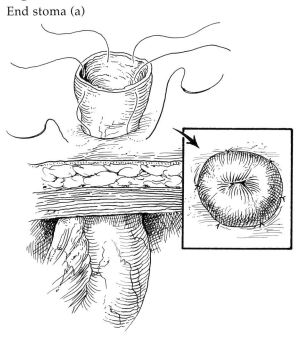

Figure 3.8
Turnbull (b)

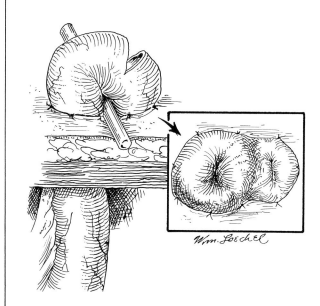

Continent Urinary Diversion to the Skin

Several techniques of continent diversion to the skin have been described [Montie et al., 1987]. They all have common principles, such as a low-pressure reservoir which is obtained by bowel detubularization, and creation of a continent mechanism to prevent leakage [Montie et al., 1987]. I will describe here the most common form of urinary diversion to the skin which we use in our service: the modified Indiana pouch [Rowland et al., 1987].

After completion of cystectomy, a segment of terminal ileum with cecum and ascending colon is isolated (Figures 3.9 and 3.10). Reanastomosis of the remaining ileum and transverse colon is accomplished by a side-to-side anastomosis using a GIA and TA-55 stapler (Figures 3.11 to 3.13). The segment of cecum, ascending colon, and ileum is thoroughly washed. Detubularization is accomplished by an anterior incision of the large bowel (Figure 3.14). The ileal segment lumen is reduced in diameter over a #14 catheter using GIA staples (Figure 3.15). The ileocecal valve is reinforced with nonabsorbable sutures to improve the continent mechanism. Prior to the folding over of the bowel, the ureters are anastomosed using the LeDuc technique [LeDuc et al., 1987] (Figure 3.16). The large bowel is folded over itself and sutured with #8 absorbable sutures (Figure 3.17). A cecostomy tube, a Foley #16 catheter, and the ureteral stents are left in place (Figure 3.18).

Figure 3.9　　Continent urinary diversion. Modified Indiana pouch; incision and bowel to be resected.

Figure 3.10　　Continent urinary diversion. Modified Indiana pouch; isolation of terminal ileum, cecum, and ascending colon.

Figure 3.11　　Continent urinary diversion. Modified Indiana pouch; using GIA stapler, the distal ileum is transected.

Figure 3.12　　Continent urinary diversion. Modified Indiana pouch; isolation and transection of transverse colon using GIA stapler.

　　　　　　　　　　　　　　　　Continent Urinary Diversion to the Skin

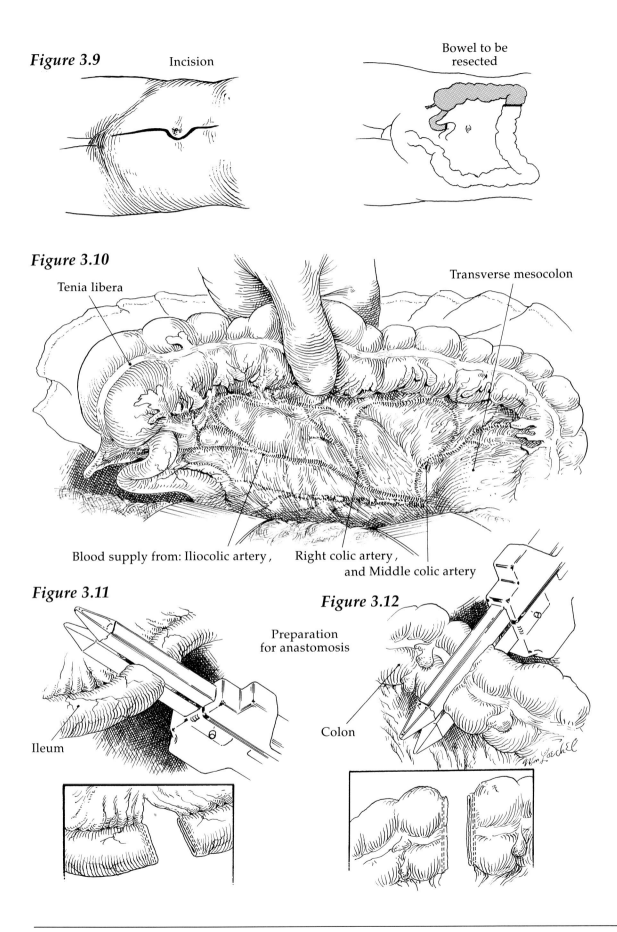

Figure 3.9   Incision

Bowel to be resected

Figure 3.10

Tenia libera

Transverse mesocolon

Blood supply from: Iliocolic artery ,   Right colic artery ,
and Middle colic artery

Figure 3.11

Figure 3.12

Preparation
for anastomosis

Ileum

Colon

Figure 3.13   Continent urinary diversion. Modified Indiana pouch; side-to-side ileocolonic anastomosis.

Figure 3.14   Continent urinary diversion. Modified Indiana pouch; anterior incision of the tenia libera to form the pouch.

Figure 3.15   Continent urinary diversion. Modified Indiana pouch; narrowing of the ileal segment over a catheter.

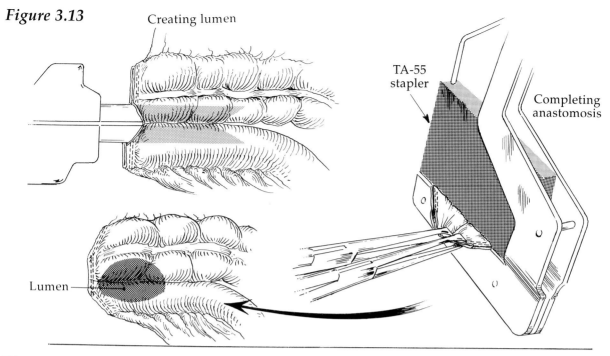

Figure 3.13

Creating lumen

TA-55 stapler

Completing anastomosis

Lumen

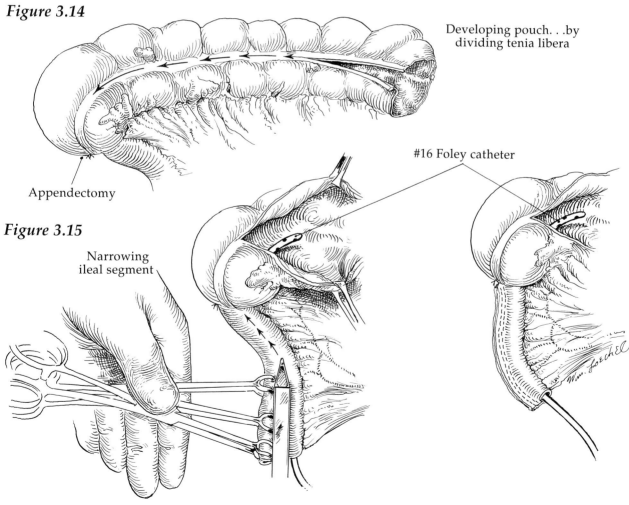

Figure 3.14

Developing pouch. . .by dividing tenia libera

Appendectomy

#16 Foley catheter

Figure 3.15

Narrowing ileal segment

Figure 3.16 *Continent urinary diversion. Modified Indiana pouch; LeDuc anastomosis of the ureters.*

Figure 3.17 *Continent urinary diversion. Modified Indiana pouch; continuous sutures of folded over bowel.*

Figure 3.18 *Continent urinary diversion. Modified Indiana pouch; completed pouch with indwelling cecostomy tube, Foley catheter, and ureteral stents.*

Continent Urinary Diversion to the Skin

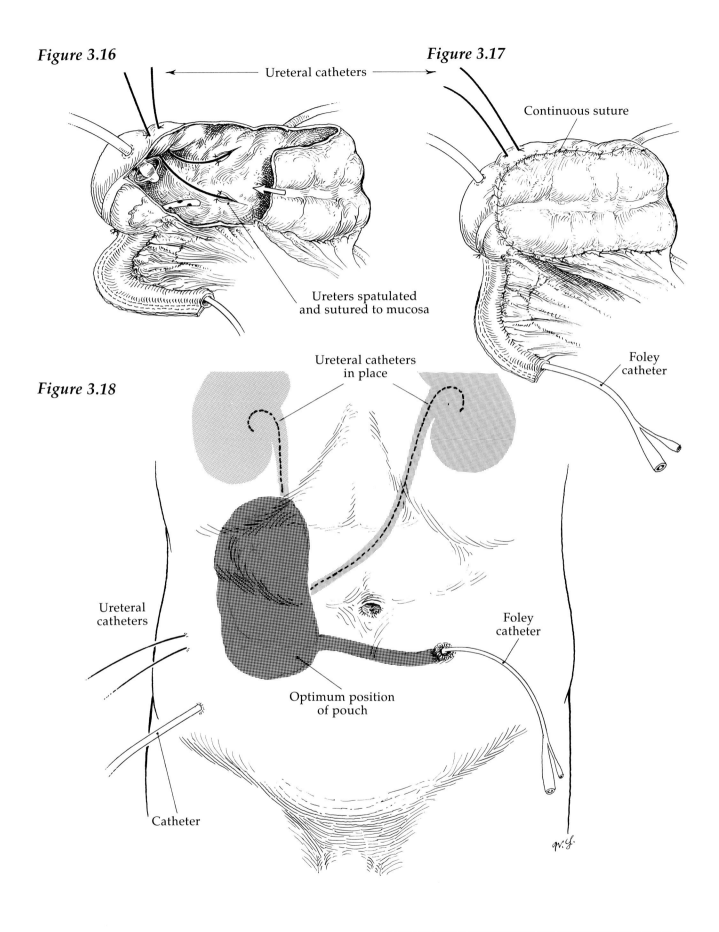

Figure 3.16

Ureteral catheters

Figure 3.17

Continuous suture

Ureters spatulated
and sutured to mucosa

Foley
catheter

Figure 3.18

Ureteral catheters
in place

Ureteral
catheters

Foley
catheter

Optimum position
of pouch

Catheter

Continent Urinary Diversion to the Urethra

Since the pioneer work of Camey, several continent urinary diversions to the urethra have been proposed [Montie et al., 1987]. The same characteristics discussed in continent diversion to the skin apply in continent diversion to the urethra. We will describe the two most commonly used diversions, the LeBag technique and W pouch [Montie et al., 1987].

LeBag Continent Urinary Diversion

A segment of cecum and ascending colon is isolated, together with a segment of terminal ileum of equal size [Light and Engelman, 1986]. Thorough washing of this isolated segment is carried out. The anastomosis between the segment of ileum and the transverse colon is done in the manner previously shown (Figures 3.11 and 3.12). An anterior incision of the ascending colon and cecum is continued into the ileal segment (Figure 3.19). After reimplantation of the ureters (Figure 3.16), the ileal segment is folded over the colon as a patch which is used to detubularize the colon (Figure 3.19). An appendectomy is performed, and the most dependent point of the cecum is reanastomosed to the urethra, which has been prepared in the same manner as for radical prostatectomy (Figure 3.20). The ureters are stented with single J catheters which are removed 7 days after surgery. A #22 Foley 5-cc catheter is left indwelling for three weeks. Irrigation at 3-hour intervals is important to prevent formation of a mucous plug.

Figure 3.19 *Continent urinary diversion. LeBag diversion; ileal segment folded over the colon.*

Figure 3.20 *Continent urinary diversion. LeBag diversion; incisions and reanastomosis.*

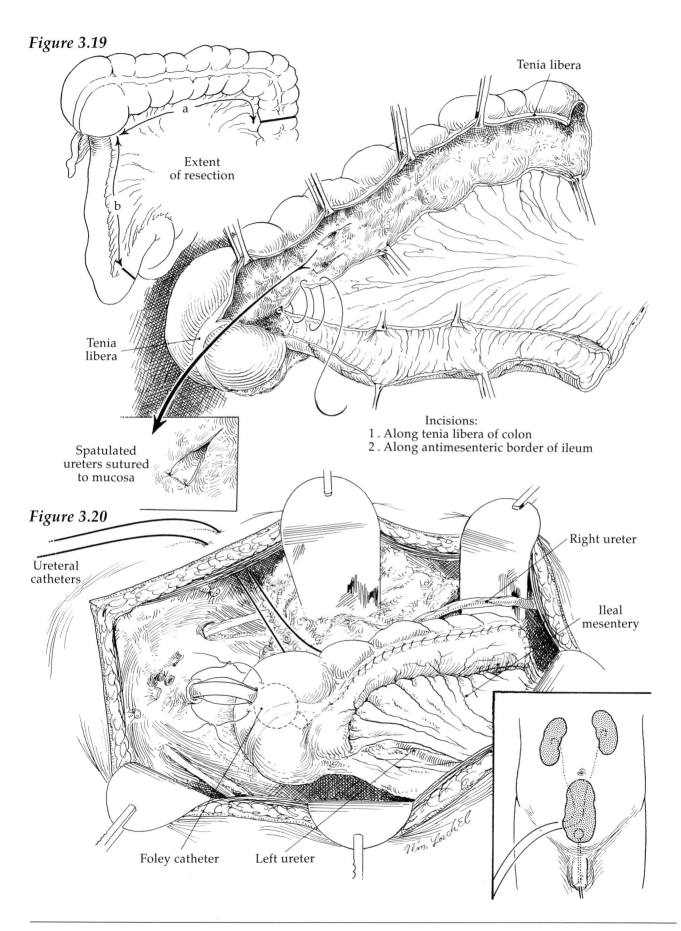

Figure 3.19

Tenia libera

Extent
of resection

Tenia
libera

Incisions:
1. Along tenia libera of colon
2. Along antimesenteric border of ileum

Spatulated
ureters sutured
to mucosa

Figure 3.20

Ureteral
catheters

Right ureter

Ileal
mesentery

Foley catheter   Left ureter

Continent Urinary Diversion to the Urethra   53

W Pouch with Absorbable Staple Anastomosis

After the bladder has been removed and four to six sutures have been placed in the urethra for later use in the urethral–neobladder anastomosis, the pelvis is prepared for creation of the reservoir. Each ureter has been mobilized, together with a large amount of periureteral adventitial tissue (Figure 3.21).

A segment of terminal ileum approximately 50 cm in length is used for the stapled W reservoir. A window is made in the mesentery on the efferent limb; the bowel is divided with a metal stapler, as depicted by the dotted line (Figure 3.22). The site of the division on the afferent limb is demonstrated in the drawing, but this is not completed until a later stage in the procedure. The most dependent portion of the W reservoir is usually the first (most distal) limb of the W (Figure 3.22).

The enterotomy is made at the apical portion of the efferent segment of the W. It is important to make the enterotomy midway between the mesentery and the opposite antimesenteric border. If the enterotomy is made directly on the antimesenteric border, the absorbable GIA staple lines are too close to the enterotomy to allow closure with the TA-55 absorbable stapler; absorbable staple lines cannot be overlapped. The poly-GIA absorbable stapler is placed in adjacent loops of bowel through the enterotomy, and firing of the stapler creates a common lumen. The inset demonstrates closure of the enterotomy with the TA-55 polysorb instrument after the endo-GIA absorbable staples have been fired (Figure 3.23).

Figure 3.21 Continent urinary diversion. W pouch; preparation of the pelvis for creation of the reservoir.

Figure 3.22 Continent urinary diversion. W pouch; division of the bowel with a metal stapler (dotted line).

Continent Urinary Diversion to the Urethra

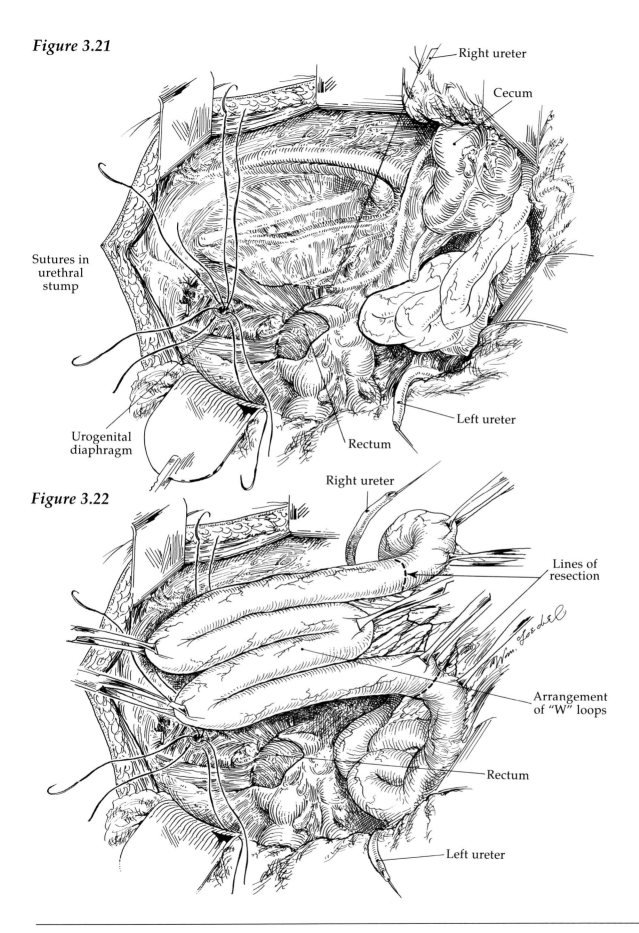

Figure 3.21

Sutures in
urethral
stump

Urogenital
diaphragm

Right ureter

Cecum

Left ureter

Rectum

Figure 3.22

Right ureter

Lines of
resection

Arrangement
of "W" loops

Rectum

Left ureter

The next step is to continue formation of the reservoir on the second limb of the W. The poly-GIA staple lines cannot be directly opposite each other because this creates a potentially ischemic segment on the anterior wall of the bowel, between the two staple lines. By staggering the staple lines, rather than having them directly opposed, the risk of ischemia can be avoided. A safe amount of overlap is in the range of 3 to 4 cm. The enterotomy is closed with the TA-55 polysorb stapler. Similarly, a third enterotomy is made on the third limb of the W, and the GIA and TA-55 staplers are fired as on the other limbs of the W (Figure 3.24).

After completion of the reservoir, a small enterotomy is made in the anterior surface of the dependent limb of the W for the urethral anastomosis. The previously placed sutures in the urethra are then placed into this enterotomy over a #22 French catheter. The ureters can be anastomosed in several different fashions depending on the surgeon's preference. Currently in use is a direct end-to-side anastomosis between the right ureter and the efferent limb and the left ureter and the afferent limb. If the surgeon's preference is for a isoperistaltic afferent limb to minimize reflux, as recommended by Studer [1992], the afferent limb can be lengthened and both ureters anastomosed to this. If the preference is for a intussuscepted nipple valve as an antireflux mechanism, as in the hemi-Kock reservoir, this can also be easily done through the third enterotomy used to make the reservoir. A LeDuc anastomosis could also be performed if desired [LeDuc et al., 1987]. Thus, there is considerable flexibility in construction of the ureteroileal anastomoses (Figure 3.25).

The enteroenterostomy is performed using metal stapling instruments and the defect in the mesentery at the site of the enteroenterostomy is closed to prevent internal herniation of the small bowel.

Figure 3.23 *Continent urinary diversion. W pouch; development of an ostium into the lumen (a) to allow stapling of adjacent loops of bowel, after which the enterotomy is closed* (inset).

Figure 3.24 *Continent urinary diversion. W pouch; formation of second and third limbs of the reservoir. Area of overlap is shown.*

Figure 3.25 *Reanastomosis between the pouch and urethra is completed.*

Figure 3.23

Developing ostia in lumina a, b, c

a

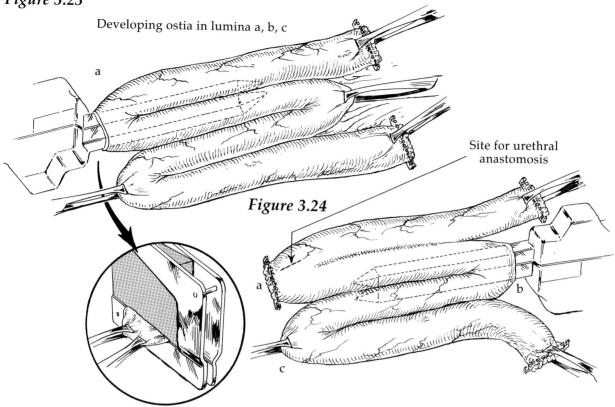

Figure 3.24

Site for urethral anastomosis

a

b

c

Figure 3.25

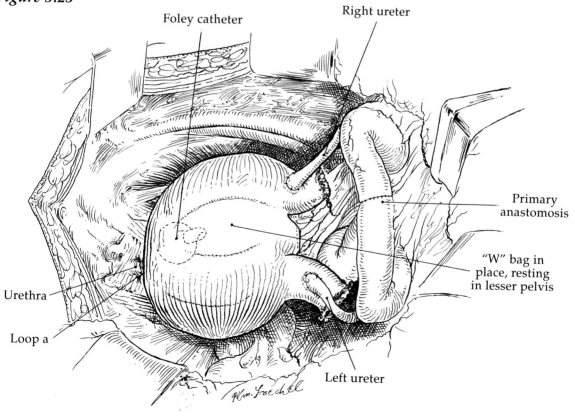

Foley catheter

Right ureter

Primary anastomosis

"W" bag in place, resting in lesser pelvis

Urethra

Loop a

Left ureter

Chapter 4

Operations for
Urinary Fistulas

Vesicovaginal Fistulas

Vesicovaginal fistulas often result from gynecological procedures. In general, the urological surgeon is consulted after one or more attempts at repair have failed. In a situation where a fistula repair has not been attempted before, it is reasonable to attempt a vaginal approach.

Vaginal Repair of Vesicovaginal Fistulas

The patient is placed in an exaggerated lithotomy position (Figure 4.1). During cystoscopic evaluation prior to surgery, if it is noted that the fistula is too close to the ureteral orifices, ureteral catheters are inserted. A weighted speculum is placed on the posterior vaginal wall. The fistula is identified anteriorly (Figure 4.2). An incision in the vaginal wall surrounding the fistula is made, and the vaginal wall is dissected free from the bladder. The fistula is excised and the bladder wall is sutured with interrupted 3-0 polyglycol sutures (Figures 4.3 and 4.4). The vaginal wall is approximated, making sure that the two lines of sutures are not superimposed.

Figure 4.1 *Vaginal repair of a vesicovaginal fistula. Exaggerated lithotomy position.*

Figure 4.2 *Vaginal repair of a vesicovaginal fistula. Anterior fistula with line of incision (dotted line).*

Figure 4.3 *Vaginal repair of a vesicovaginal fistula. Vertical closure of bladder wall defect and fascia.*

Figure 4.4 *Vaginal repair of a vesicovaginal fistula. Horizontal closure of vaginal wall defect.*

Vesicovaginal Fistulas

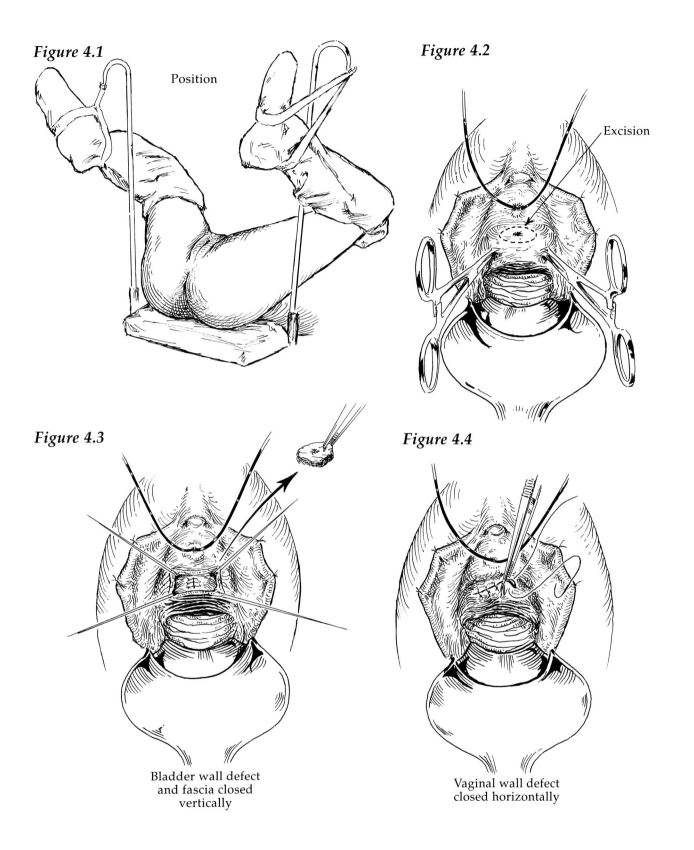

Figure 4.1

Position

Figure 4.2

Excision

Figure 4.3

Bladder wall defect
and fascia closed
vertically

Figure 4.4

Vaginal wall defect
closed horizontally

Abdominal Repair of Vesicovaginal Fistulas

Vesicovaginal fistulas of difficult repair are better approached abdominally. A technique which has been used successfully for many years is the one described by O'Connor [1979]. A vertical midline intraperitoneal incision is used (Figure 4.5). I find it helpful during the vaginal preparation to leave a roll in the vagina to help in the dissection of the bladder from the anterior vaginal wall. After the bladder is dissected from the surrounding tissues, it is opened and bivalved posteriorly to the area of the fistula (Figure 4.6). The area of the fistula is completely excised from the normal bladder (Figure 4.7). The vaginal defect is identified and repaired (Figure 4.8). The bladder is closed in two layers: a muscular layer, using 2-0 polyglycol; and mucosal layer, using 4-0 polyglycol sutures (Figure 4.8). To assure adequate drainage of urine and that there is no pressure over the repaired area, a simple catheter with a nylon string coming out of the abdomen wall and a Malecot type of suprapubic catheter is used.

A variation of the above technique has been described previously and is helpful when multiple repairs have been attempted and difficulties are encountered in liberating the bladder from the vagina [Pontes, 1974]. The bladder is opened and the fistula identified (Figure 4.9). The fistula is resected, but no attempt is made to dissect the surrounding tissues (Figure 4.9). A flap from the mobile part of the lateral wall of the bladder is isolated (Figure 4.9), and the flap is advanced to cover the defect (Figure 4.10). Urinary drainage is provided as shown in Figure 4.11.

Figure 4.5 Abdominal repair of a vesicovaginal fistula (inset). Vertical midline intraperitoneal incision.

Figure 4.6 Abdominal repair of a vesicovaginal fistula. Opened dome of the bladder.

Figure 4.7 Abdominal repair of a vesicovaginal fistula. Complete excision of the fistula.

Figure 4.8 Abdominal repair of a vesicovaginal fistula. Identification and repair of vaginal defect (left, a) is followed by bladder closure (left, b) and insertion of catheters (right).

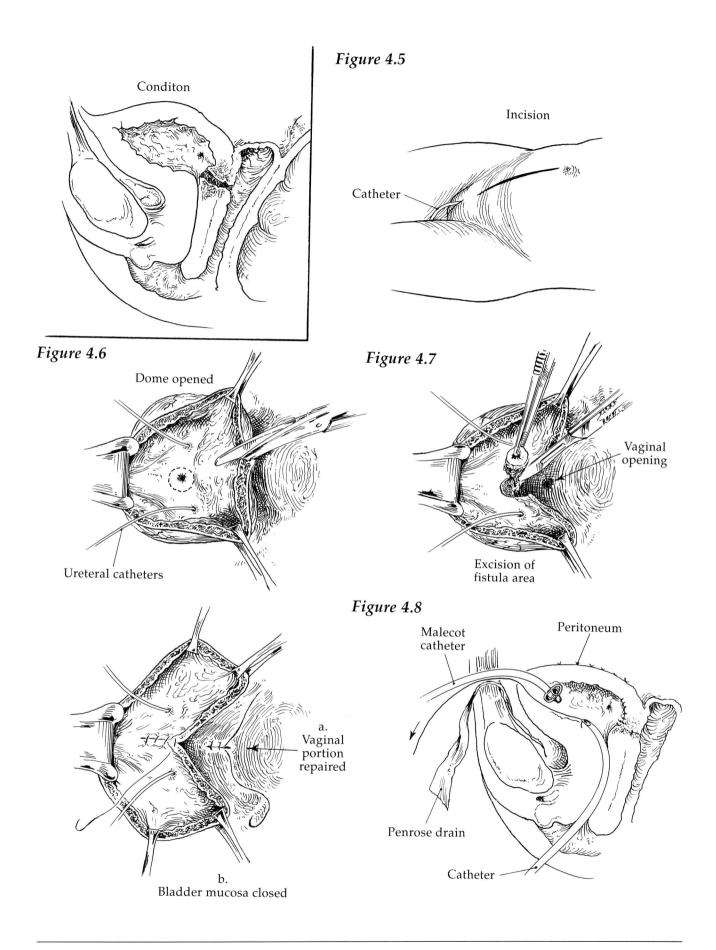

Figure 4.5

Conditon

Incision

Catheter

Figure 4.6

Dome opened

Ureteral catheters

Figure 4.7

Vaginal opening

Excision of fistula area

Figure 4.8

Malecot catheter

Peritoneum

a. Vaginal portion repaired

Penrose drain

b. Bladder mucosa closed

Catheter

Figure 4.9   *Abdominal repair of a vesicovaginal fistula. Fistula excision and isolation of a flap from the lateral wall of the bladder.*

Figure 4.10   *Abdominal repair of a vesicovaginal fistula. The bladder flap is advanced to cover the defect.*

Figure 4.11   *Abdominal repair of a vesicovaginal fistula. Urinary drainage.*

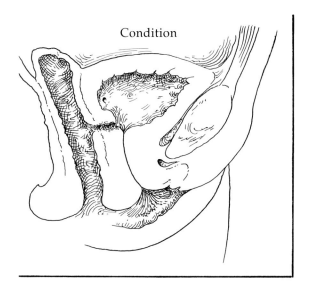

Condition

Figure 4.9

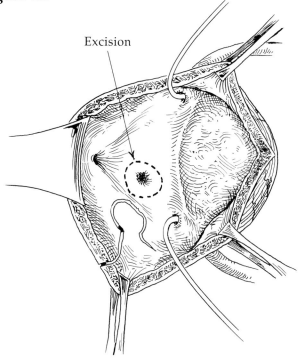

Excision

Figure 4.10

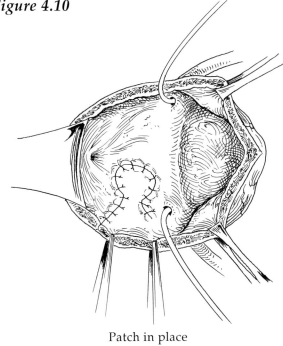

Patch in place

Figure 4.11

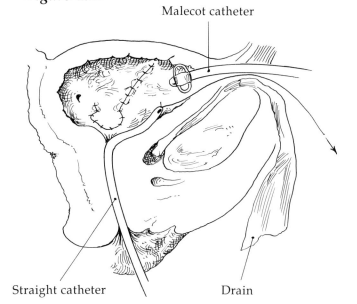

Malecot catheter

Straight catheter

Drain

Vesicoenteric Fistulas

Vesicoenteric fistulas can result either from inflammatory or neoplastic conditions. In the case illustrated, a sigmoid tumor has invaded the dome of the bladder (Figure 4.12). Procedures for such tumors are usually carried out in consultation with colorectal surgeons to minimize morbidity. A long, vertical midline incision is used (Figure 4.13). The left colon and the sigmoid colon above and below the involved area are isolated (Figure 4.14). The area of bladder involvement is identified and isolated from surrounding tissues (Figure 4.14). Resection of the sigmoid colon and the area of the bladder involving the tumor is performed (Figure 4.15). The same care is taken in obtaining negative tumor margins as in the case of partial cystectomy (Chapter 2). The bowel is reanastomosed and the bladder closed in two layers (Figure 4.16). The decision regarding a temporary colostomy depends on the general nutrition of the patient and whether the procedure was done on an emergency or elective basis. The interposition of omentum between the bladder repair and the colon should be considered, depending on intraoperative factors.

Figure 4.12   *Vesicoenteric fistula. Sigmoid tumor invading the dome of the bladder.*

Figure 4.13   *Vesicoenteric fistula. Vertical midline incision.*

Figure 4.14   *Vesicoenteric fistula. Isolation of the bladder area involved from surrounding tissues; excision of the colon between clamps.*

Figure 4.12

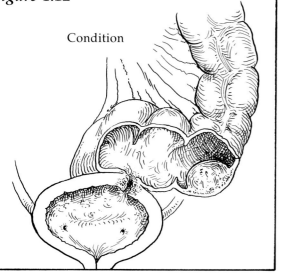

Condition

Figure 4.13

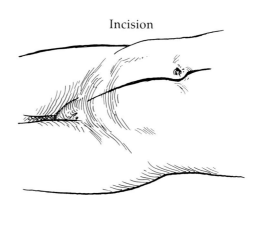

Incision

Figure 4.14

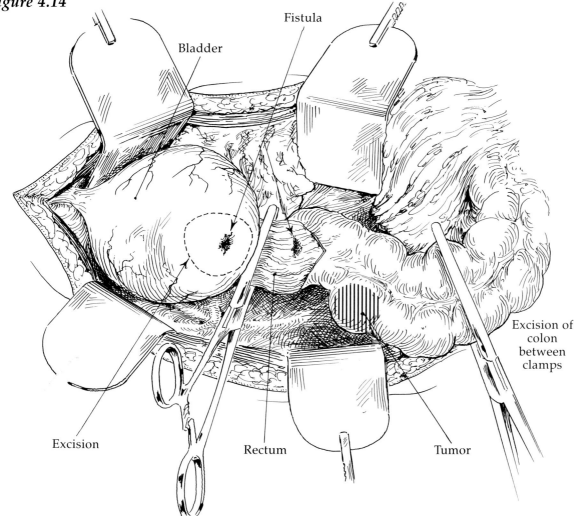

Bladder

Fistula

Excision

Rectum

Tumor

Excision of colon between clamps

Figure 4.15   *Vesicoenteric fistula. Resection of the sigmoid colon and bladder area involved to yield the specimen shown* (left).

Figure 4.16   *Vesicoenteric fistula. Bowel reanastomosis and bladder closure.*

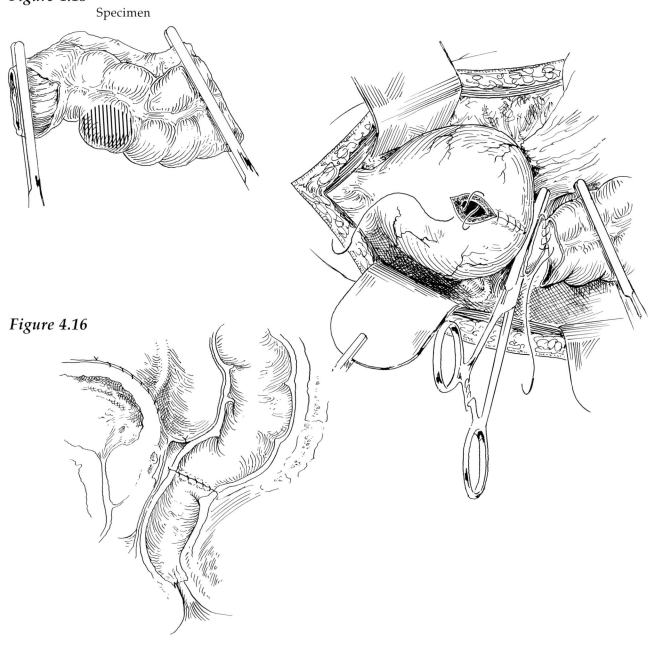

Figure 4.15

Specimen

Figure 4.16

The Use of the Omentum Flap

In many situations it is desirable to interpose omentum after excision and repair of vesicovaginal or vesicoenteric fistulas [Pierce, 1989]. The most common technique uses the gastroepiploic artery as the main blood supply for the flap. The omentum is separated from the transverse colon by sharp dissection. The short gastric arteries are individually ligated and the omentum is liberated (Figure 4.17). The omentum is brought down to the pelvis either by the paracolic gutter or, as shown here, through windows in the mesocolon and mesentery. Interposition between the fistula repair and the vagina will aid in healing.

Figure 4.17 *Vesicoenteric fistula. Omentum flap, in which the mobilized omentum is passed through the transverse mesocolon.*

Figure 4.17

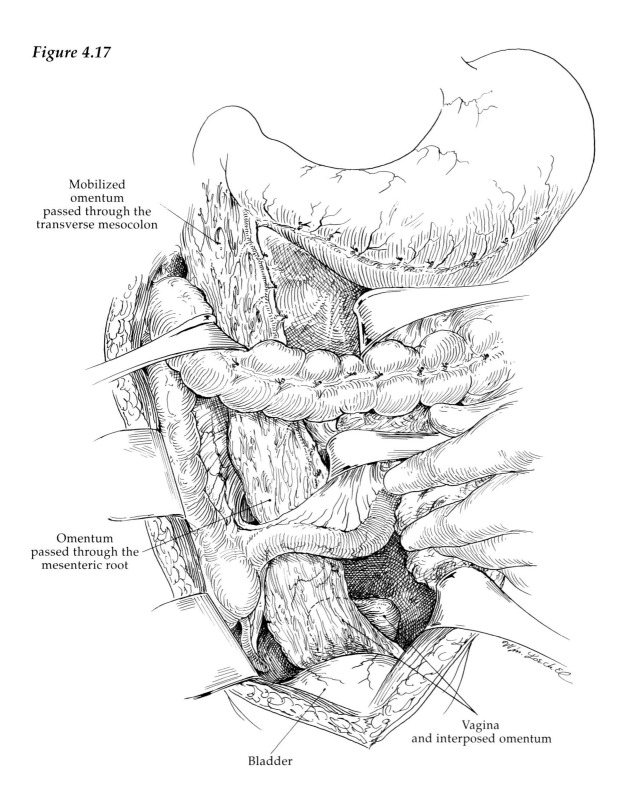

Mobilized
omentum
passed through the
transverse mesocolon

Omentum
passed through the
mesenteric root

Vagina
and interposed omentum

Bladder

Chapter 5

Radical Prostatectomy

Radical prostatectomy has become the most frequently used form of therapy for patients with localized prostate cancer. Although this procedure can be done perineally or retropubically, the perineal approach is used only in a minority of institutions in the United States. The resurgence of radical prostatectomy has been largely due to the work of Walsh and associates [1983]. A variation of their technique, as modified by the author, is described here [Pontes, 1989]. A vertical midline incision is used (Figure 5.1) and by sharp and blunt dissection the bladder and surrounding peritoneum are freed. A self-retained retractor is used. The procedure starts with a modified pelvic lymphadenectomy (Figure 5.2). All the areolar tissue in an area medial to the external iliac artery, including nodal tissue around the obturator nerve, is removed. The obturator vessels may be saved, or sacrificed as shown in Figure 5.3. The area of this modified pelvic lymphadenectomy is as shown in Figure 5.4.

Figure 5.1 *Radical prostatectomy. Vertical midline incision.*

Figure 5.2 *Radical prostatectomy. Modified pelvic lymphadenectomy.*

Figure 5.3 *Radical prostatectomy. Sacrifice of obturator vessels.*

Figure 5.4 *Radical prostatectomy. Area of modified lymphadenectomy.*

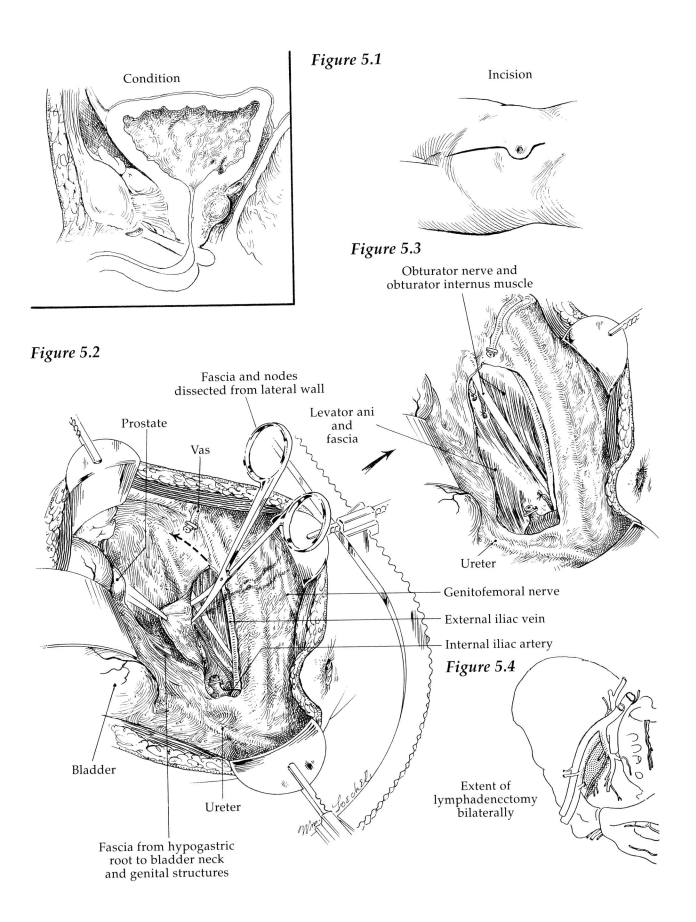

Figure 5.1

Condition

Incision

Figure 5.3

Obturator nerve and
obturator internus muscle

Figure 5.2

Fascia and nodes
dissected from lateral wall

Prostate

Vas

Levator ani
and
fascia

Genitofemoral nerve

External iliac vein

Internal iliac artery

Ureter

Bladder

Ureter

Figure 5.4

Extent of
lymphadenectomy
bilaterally

Fascia from hypogastric
root to bladder neck
and genital structures

The position of the patient for the radical prostatectomy is shown in Figure 5.5. A flat bag under the sacrum provides hyperextension which is important during the apical portion of the dissection of the prostate (Figure 5.5). The endopelvic fascia is opened bilaterally, the puboprostatic ligaments are transected, and the dorsal vein of the penis complex is ligated using a 5/8 needle with 2-0 polyglycol suture (Figure 5.6). The urethra is transected and the Foley catheter is used as a tractor to aid in the dissection of the prostate from the rectum (Figures 5.7 and 5.8). Prior to the completion of the transection of the urethra, two sutures are placed at the eleven o'clock and one o'clock positions. This will aid later in the placement of the posterior sutures.

Figure 5.5   *Radical prostatectomy. Placement of a flat bag under the sacrum to provide hyperextension.*

Figure 5.6   *Radical prostatectomy. Opening of the endopelvic fascia, transection of the puboprostatic ligaments, and ligation of the dorsal vein of the penis complex.*

Figure 5.7   *Radical prostatectomy. Transection of the urethra.*

Figure 5.8   *Radical prostatectomy. Retrograde dissection. The Foley catheter is used as a tractor to aid in separating the prostate from the rectum.*

Radical Prostatectomy

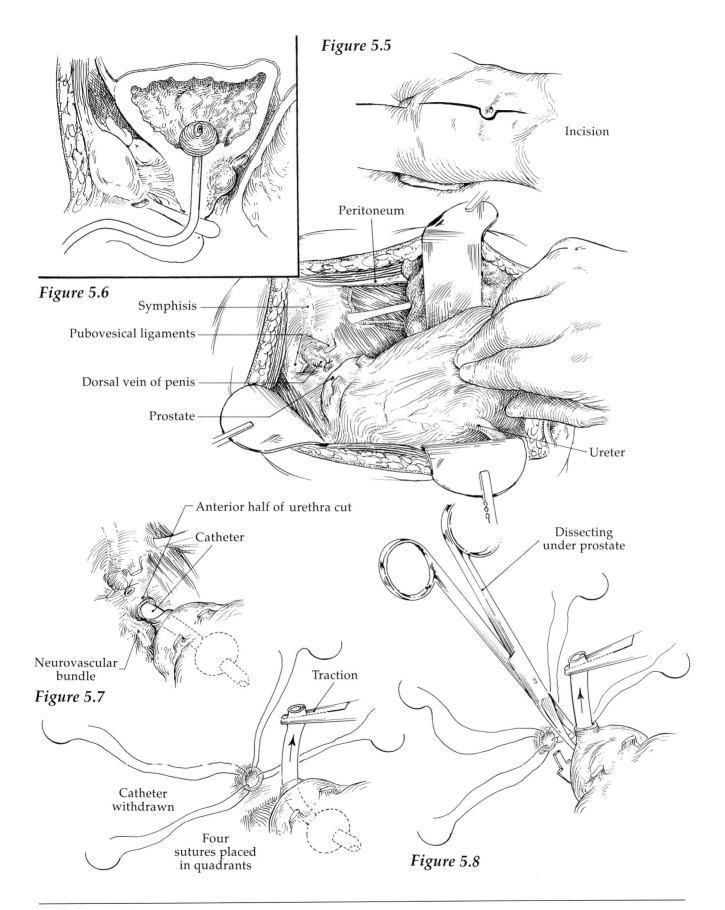

Figure 5.5

Incision

Peritoneum

Figure 5.6

Symphisis

Pubovesical ligaments

Dorsal vein of penis

Prostate

Ureter

Dissecting under prostate

Anterior half of urethra cut

Catheter

Neurovascular bundle

Figure 5.7

Traction

Catheter withdrawn

Four sutures placed in quadrants

Figure 5.8

Radical Prostatectomy

The retrograde dissection of the prostate from the rectum is started by using a special pair of right-angle scissors to divide the rectourethralis muscle and develop a midline plane between the prostate and the rectum (Figure 5.9). The vessels in the lateral pedicles of the prostate are controlled either by coagulation or the use of metal clips. In selected cases, by transecting the pedicles close to the prostate, the neurovascular bundles are preserved. After the retrograde dissection of the prostate from the rectum is completed, a anterograde approach is used with transection of the bladder neck (Figure 5.9). An incision is made between the base of the prostate and the Foley balloon (Figure 5.9). By using scissors, the bladder neck is separated from the prostate while preserving the circular fibers. After the transection of the bladder neck, the Foley catheter is folded back to form a loop and the ampullae of the vas deferens are visualized at the midline. Ligation of the ampullae of the vas deferens, and the final dissection of the seminal vesicles are accomplished (Figure 5.10).

I often use a posterior incision of Denovilliers' fascia to achieve the proper plane of dissection of the seminal vesicles posteriorly (Figure 5.11). Reduction in the diameter of the bladder neck is done, if necessary. The bladder mucosa is approximated over the bladder neck using 4-0 polyglycol sutures to prevent late stricture. A reanastomosis is completed between the bladder neck and urethra using the four sutures previously placed in the urethra over a #22 Foley catheter with a 5-cc balloon (Figure 5.12). Two closed drainage drains (JP) are left in the area of the lymph node dissection and are removed when the drainage falls below 60 to 80 ml in 24 hours. A Foley catheter is left indwelling for three weeks from the day of surgery.

Figure 5.9   *Radical prostatectomy. Retrograde dissection of the prostrate from the rectum (right); anterior dissection starting with transection of the bladder neck (left).*

Figure 5.10   *Radical prostatectomy. Anterior dissection: incision between the base of the prostate and the Foley balloon; folding back of the Foley catheter to form a loop; ligation of the ampullae of the vas deferens; dissection of the seminal vesicles.*

Figure 5.11   *Radical prostatectomy. Plane of dissection obtained by posterior incision of Denonvilliers' fascia.*

Figure 5.12   *Radical prostatectomy. Reanastomosis between the bladder neck and the urethra.*

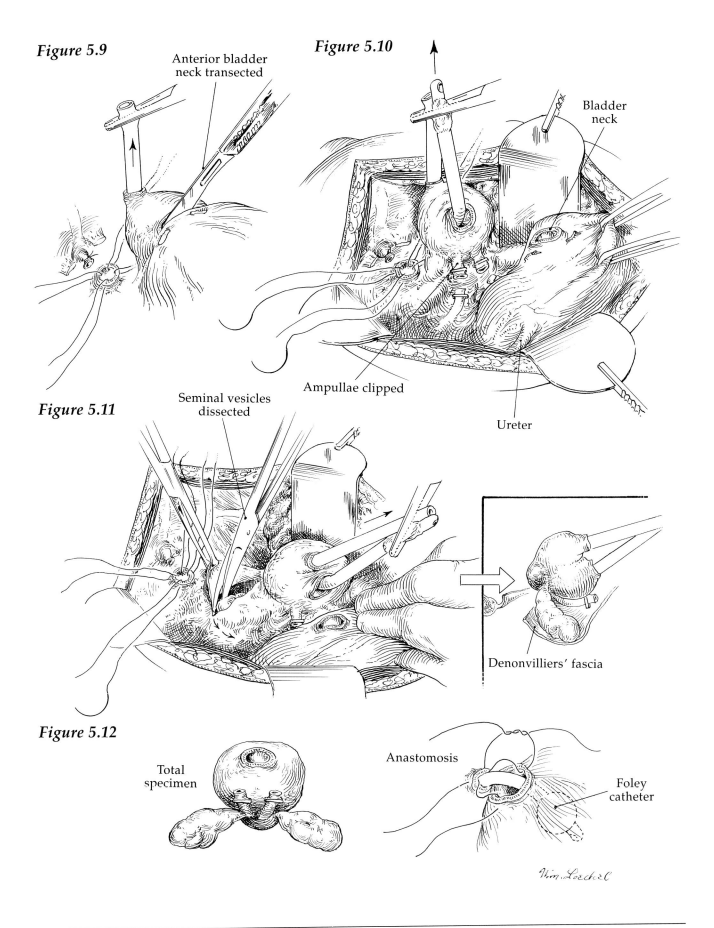

Figure 5.9

Anterior bladder neck transected

Figure 5.10

Bladder neck

Ampullae clipped

Ureter

Figure 5.11

Seminal vesicles dissected

Denonvilliers' fascia

Figure 5.12

Total specimen

Anastomosis

Foley catheter

Nim. Loechel

Chapter 6

Surgery for Penile and Urethral Cancers

Penile and Urethral Cancers

Penile cancers are uncommon in Western countries [Pontes, 1992]. Because of this, urological surgeons may not be as familiar with the surgical management of this condition as they are for treating other, more frequent cancers. An illustration of the different layers of the penis with the fascia and vascular supply is shown in Figure 6.1. Illustrated in this figure is the superficial dorsal vein of the penis and its relation to Colles' fascia and to the deep fascia of the penis (Buck's fascia).

Penile cancers which can be treated by partial penectomy include those that can be excised with a 2-cm free margin beyond the tumor and with enough penile length to preserve a functional organ [Bissada, 1992]. A tourniquet is applied to the base of the penis to decrease bleeding. The tumor is covered with a condom catheter to prevent contamination of the wound (Figure 6.2). A circular incision through the skin, Colles' and Buck's fasciae, and the corpora cavernosa is made 2 cm proximal to the tumor (Figure 6.3). The urethra is sectioned separately 0.5 cm distal to the circular incision (Figure 6.4). The urethra is spatulated to prevent future stenosis and the corpora are ligated en bloc with 2-0 polyglycol sutures (Figure 6.4). The skin will cover the defect and it is approximated over the spatulated urethra (Figure 6.5).

Figure 6.1 *Layers of the penis, showing the fascia and blood supply.*

Figure 6.2 *Partial penectomy. Tourniquet and condom catheter.*

Figure 6.3 *Partial penectomy. Circular incision through the skin, Colles' and Buck's fasciae, and the corpora cavernosa.*

Figure 6.4 *Partial penectomy. Section and spatulation of the urethra; closure of the corpora cavernosa.*

Figure 6.5 *Partial penectomy. Closure: the skin covers the defect and approximates over the urethra.*

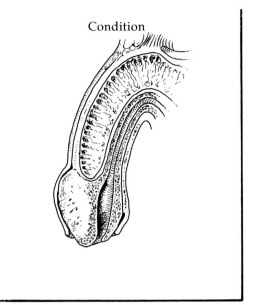
Condition

Figure 6.1

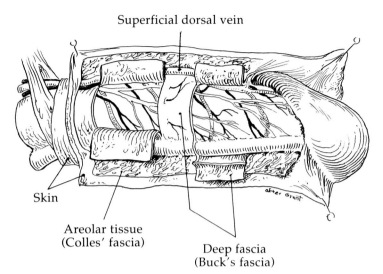

Superficial dorsal vein

Skin

Areolar tissue
(Colles' fascia)

Deep fascia
(Buck's fascia)

Figure 6.2

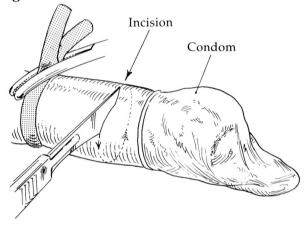

Incision

Condom

Figure 6.3

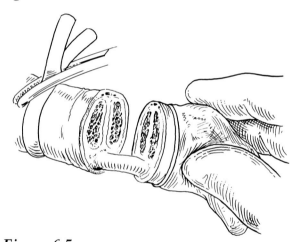

Figure 6.4

Closing corpora

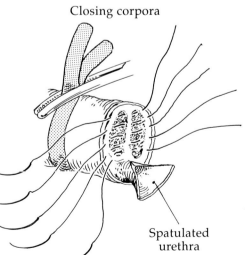

Spatulated
urethra

Figure 6.5

Closure

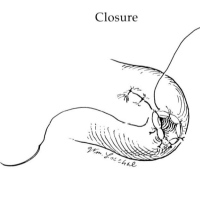

When the tumor invades the shaft of the penis and/or is too extensive for partial excision, a total penectomy is indicated. The incision used is a circular incision in the base of the penis with a vertical extension over the pubis (Figure 6.6). After dissection of the areolar tissue, the suspensory ligament is identified and transected (Figure 6.7). This will improve access to the corpora cavernosa which are dissected to their insertion at the ischium. By mobilizing the penis upwards, its ventral surface is exposed, and dissection and transection of the urethral stump is done (Figure 6.8). Stay sutures are placed in the urethra, and the corpora are ventrally dissected to their ischial insertion, and excised (Figure 6.9).

A semicircular incision is made in the perineum at the base of the scrotum and the urethra is brought into this position as a perineal urethrostomy (Figures 6.10 and 6.11). The anterior incision is closed and drained (Figure 6.12). The perineal incision is closed and a Foley catheter is left indwelling for five to seven days (Figure 6.13).

Figure 6.6   Total penectomy. Circular incision with extension over the pubis.

Figure 6.7   Total penectomy. Transection of the suspensory ligament.

Figure 6.8   Total penectomy. Transection of the urethral stump.

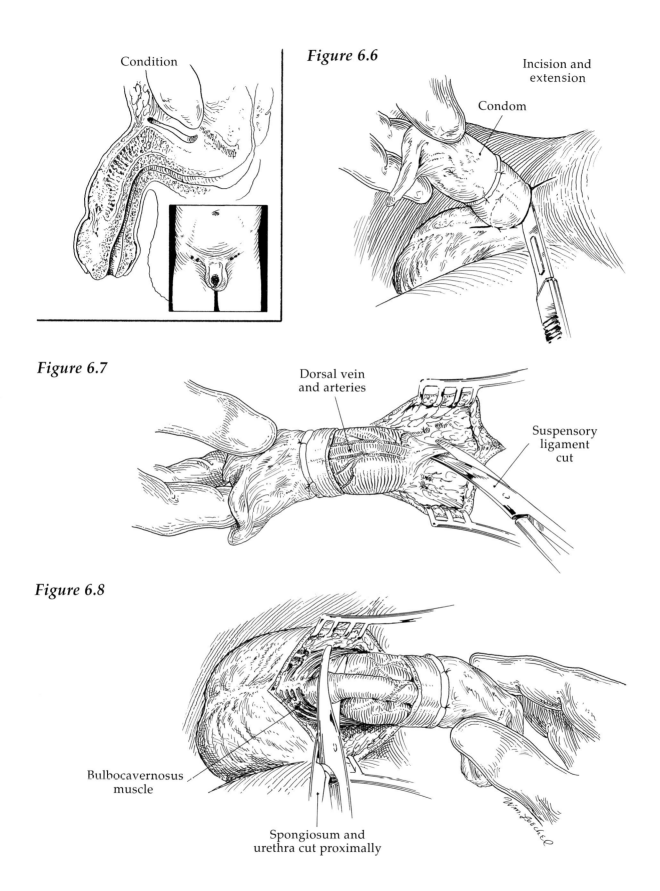

Condition

Figure 6.6

Incision and
extension

Condom

Figure 6.7

Dorsal vein
and arteries

Suspensory
ligament
cut

Figure 6.8

Bulbocavernosus
muscle

Spongiosum and
urethra cut proximally

Figure 6.9   *Total penectomy. Placement of stay sutures and excision of*
               the corpora cavernosa.

Figure 6.10   *Total penectomy. Perineal urethrostomy: a passing clamp*
and   *brings the urethra into position through a semicircular incision*
Figure 6.11   *in the perineum at the base of the scrotum.*

Figure 6.12   *Total penectomy. Closure and drainage of the anterior incision.*

Figure 6.13   *Total penectomy. Closure of the perineal incision.*

Penile and Urethral Cancers

Figure 6.9

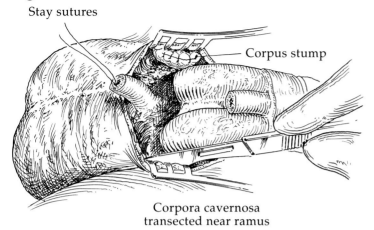

Stay sutures

Corpus stump

Corpora cavernosa
transected near ramus

Figure 6.10

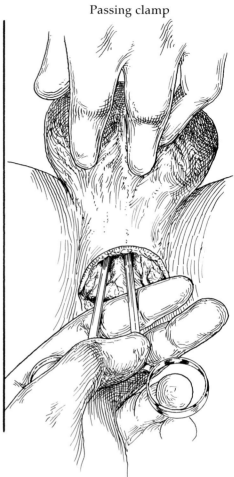

Passing clamp

Figure 6.11

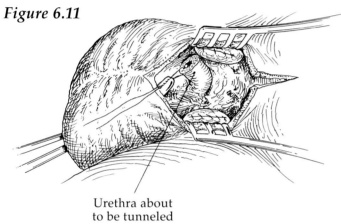

Urethra about
to be tunneled

Figure 6.13

Figure 6.12

Pubic closure

Perineal closure

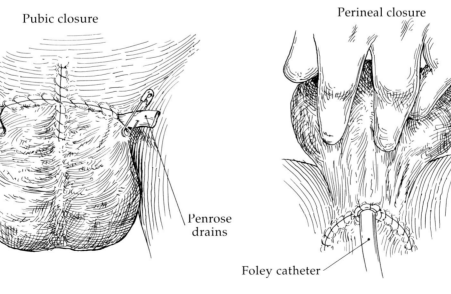

Penrose
drains

Foley catheter

Superficial Inguinal Node Dissection

The indications for superficial inguinal node dissections for patients with penile cancer have been the subject of several publications, including recent reviews [Abi-Aad and DeKernion, 1992; Pontes, 1992].

Illustrated in this chapter is a patient who, following total penectomy and an appropriate course of antibiotic therapy, still has a palpable inguinal lymph node. The position of the patient with external rotation of the thighs is illustrated (Figure 6.14). I use a slightly curved incision below the inguinal ligament because after undermining both the skin flaps one gets better exposure to the lower area of the femoral triangle by using a semicircular incision (Figure 6.15). The skin is dissected away from the underlying areolar tissue, while preserving Camper's fascia to prevent flap necrosis (Figure 6.16). A truncated triangle, with the base at the inguinal ligament and the apex of the distal part of the femoral triangle, outlines the area of dissection. In the past, most surgeons would start the node dissection with the ligation of the great saphenous vein at the apex of this triangle, and remove it where it enters the femoral vein, together with the nodal tissue. In order to decrease edema, most authors today advocate, when possible, preservation of this vein. The area of dissection is outlined (Figure 6.17).

An incision is made in the fascia lata with removal of all the areolar tissue, including the nodal tissue behind the entrance of the great saphenous vein into the femoral vein (Figure 6.17). This will leave exposed the femoral artery and vein (Figure 6.18). To cover these structures the sartorius muscle is transected near its insertion in the superior iliac crest and transposed to the inguinal ligament (Figure 6.19). The wound is closed with a fine 4-0 nylon and left with a small closed-system drain and mild compression dressing.

Figure 6.14   *Superficial inguinal node dissection. Position of patient.*

Figure 6.15   *Superficial inguinal node dissection. Semicircular incision.*

Figure 6.16   *Superficial inguinal node dissection. Dissection of skin from underlying areolar tissue.*

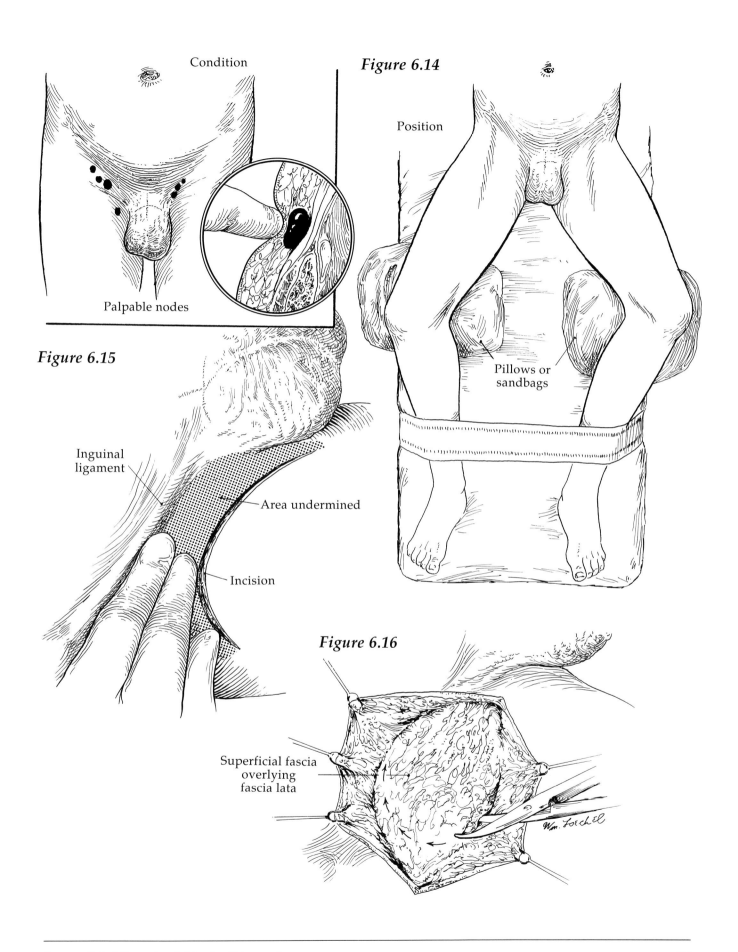

Condition

Figure 6.14

Position

Palpable nodes

Pillows or
sandbags

Figure 6.15

Inguinal
ligament

Area undermined

Incision

Figure 6.16

Superficial fascia
overlying
fascia lata

Wm. Loechel

Superficial Inguinal Node Dissection

Figure 6.17   *Superficial inguinal node dissection. Incision in the fascia lata. Lifting of nodal tissue, exposure of femoral artery and vein.*

Figure 6.18   *Superficial inguinal node dissection. Exposure of the femoral artery and vein. Transection of the sartorius muscle.*

Figure 6.19   *Superficial inguinal node dissection. Transposition of the sartorius muscle.*

Figure 6.17

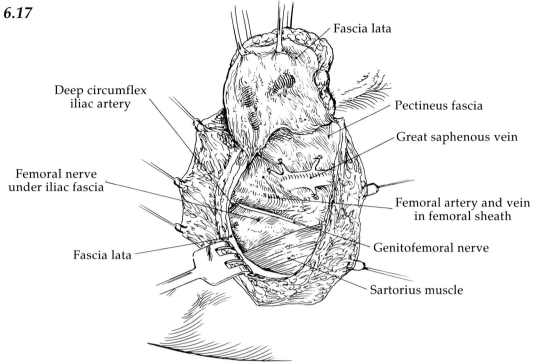

Fascia lata

Deep circumflex
iliac artery

Pectineus fascia

Great saphenous vein

Femoral nerve
under iliac fascia

Femoral artery and vein
in femoral sheath

Genitofemoral nerve

Fascia lata

Sartorius muscle

Figure 6.18

Figure 6.19

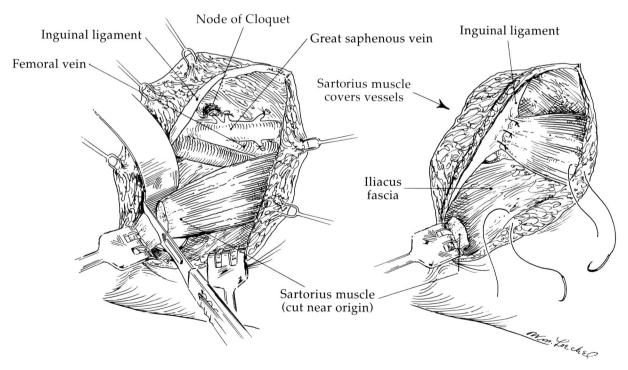

Inguinal ligament

Node of Cloquet

Great saphenous vein

Inguinal ligament

Femoral vein

Sartorius muscle
covers vessels

Iliacus
fascia

Sartorius muscle
(cut near origin)

Superficial Inguinal Node Dissection

Surgery for Local Tumor Recurrence of the Superficial Inguinal Region

Tumors which metastasize to the superficial inguinal area are treated usually by superficial inguinal node dissection (discussed earlier). On occasion, either because of incomplete resection resulting in local recurrence or failure of radiation to control the disease, or in cases with very advanced tumors, a wide excision of the tumor mass, including the skin, must be carried out, and necessitates a myocutaneous flap to cover the defect. In the case illustrated here, a urethral carcinoma which had metastasized to the inguinal nodes was unsuccessfully treated by radiation therapy (Figure 6.20). A wide excision of the area beyond the noted radiation changes is necessary (Figure 6.21). The underlying fat is dissected from the muscular layer (Figure 6.22). The tumor mass is dissected en bloc from the area behind the entrance of the saphenous vein into the femoral vein (Figure 6.23). Isolation and identification of the femoral artery and vein is shown in Figure 6.23. The inguinal ligament often has to be partially excised. The specimen is removed and is comprised of skin, areolar tissue, and nodes (Figure 6.24). The resulting defect has to be covered by a myocutaneous flap, and the choice of the flaps is decided by the plastic surgeon member of the team. In this illustration, the defect has been covered during the development of the fascia lata flap (Figure 6.25).

Figure 6.20   Urethral carcinoma metastasis to the inguinal nodes.

Figure 6.21   Metastatic urethral carcinoma. Wide excision.

Figure 6.22   Metastatic urethral carcinoma. Dissection of fat from the muscular layer.

Figure 6.23   Metastatic urethral carcinoma. Dissection of tumor mass en bloc; isolation of the femoral artery and vein.

Figure 6.24   Metastatic urethral carcinoma. Specimen, showing nodes.

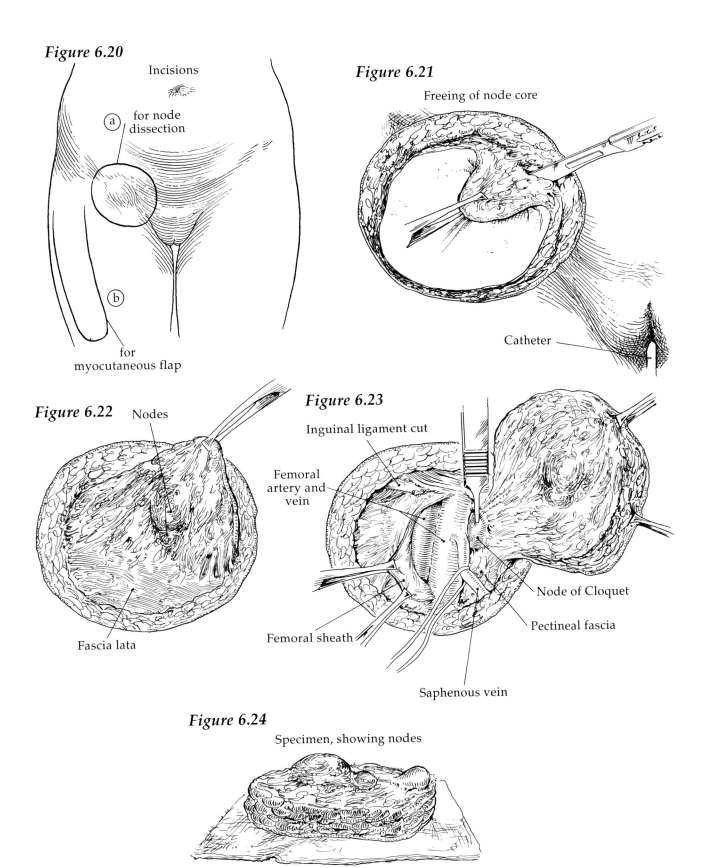

Figure 6.20

Incisions

ⓐ for node dissection

ⓑ for myocutaneous flap

Figure 6.21

Freeing of node core

Catheter

Figure 6.22 Nodes

Fascia lata

Figure 6.23

Inguinal ligament cut

Femoral artery and vein

Femoral sheath

Node of Cloquet

Pectineal fascia

Saphenous vein

Figure 6.24

Specimen, showing nodes

The availability of flaps, either from the abdominal wall or especially from the thigh, changes and depends on the size and the cause of the defect. Gracilis, sartorius, rectus femoris, vastus lateralis, and tensor fasciae latae are accessible from the thigh for reconstruction. Rectus abdominis as a muscle alone or as a muscle skin combination is probably the premium tissue source which can be obtained from the abdominal wall. With respect to their volume, blood supply, and versatility, the tensor fasciae latae and the rectus abdominis muscles are the most reliable and applicable flaps for the reconstruction of the groin defects.

Tensor Fasciae Latae Flap

This musculocutaneous flap has a small, thin, flat muscle component but has a large proximal dominant blood supply and a broad extension of fasciae distally. This anatomical advantage facilitates elevation of an area of skin measuring 8 × 40 cm from the lateral two-thirds of the thigh.

The blood supply is based on the lateral circumflex femoral branch of the deep femoral artery. This dominant blood supply enters the muscle 8 to 10 cm below the anterior iliac spine. The distal two-thirds of the faciae are supplied by a few perforators which can all be divided without any risk, during the elevation of the flap.

The flap is elevated in the distal to proximal direction (Figure 6.25). The fascia lata is sutured to the overlying skin island during the elevation of the flap. This will minimize the ischemic insult to the flap by preventing the disruption of the perforators. The vascular pedicle is identified over the medial aspects of the muscle and protected. The flap then can be transferred to the groin defect and sutured to its new location (Figure 6.26). The donor defect over the lateral aspect of the thigh can be closed primarily in most of the instances (Figure 6.27). Occasionally grafting may be necessary if a large cutaneous territory is required for the reconstruction.

Figure 6.25   *Tensor fasciae latae flap. Incision.*

Figure 6.26   *Tensor fasciae latae flap. Transfer and suture to the groin.*

Figure 6.27   *Tensor fasciae latae flap. Primary closure of donor area.*

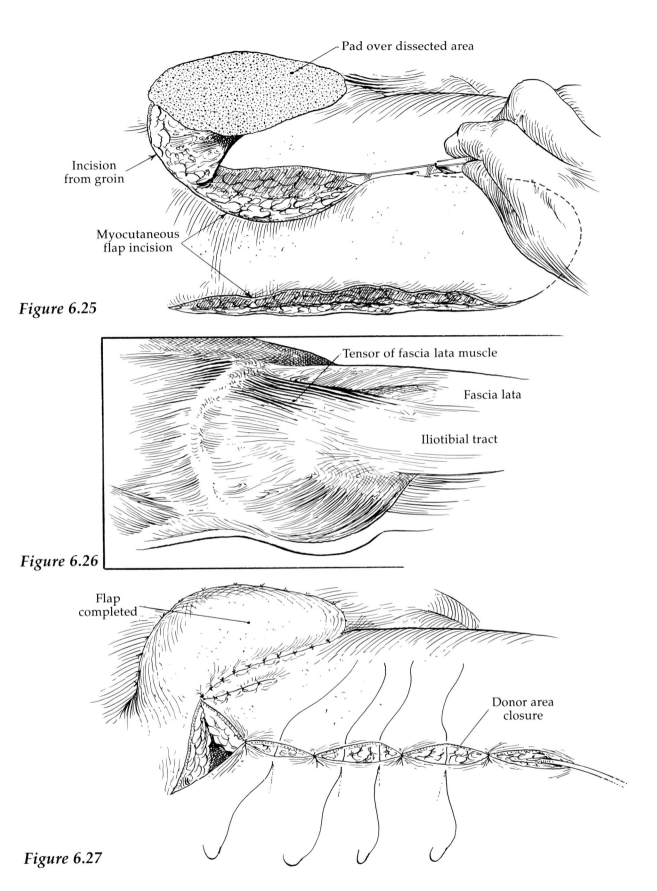

Pad over dissected area

Incision
from groin

Myocutaneous
flap incision

Figure 6.25

Tensor of fascia lata muscle

Fascia lata

Iliotibial tract

Figure 6.26

Flap
completed

Donor area
closure

Figure 6.27

Rectus Abdominis Flap

The rectus abdominis muscles are paired anterior paramedian muscles of the abdominal wall. Rectus sheet covers the muscle along its entire length, except below the arcuate line posteriorly. The rectus muscles lie only on the fasciae transversalis inferior to this line. The dual blood supply is from the inferior and superior epigastric arteries. Musculocutaneous perforators emerge in greater consistency over the paraumbilical region (Figure 6.28). The entire flap can survive on either pedicle. Obviously, the muscle should be based on the ipsilateral inferior epigastric artery for coverage of the groin defects. The vascular pedicle can be observed behind the rectus muscle entering it at the level of the umbilicus (Figure 6.28). Flap design and dimensions depend on the demand for coverage (Figure 6.29). Elevation of the flap requires a segment of rectus muscle and its anterior rectus sheath that contains the consistent perforators emerging from the muscle.

The distal end of the flap is elevated first while ensuring preservation of the important areolar tissue and the subcutaneous fat. This is essential for maintaining the optimum blood supply to the cutaneous portion of the flap (Figure 6.30). The rectus muscle with its cutaneous island is raised together with the anterior rectus sheath (Figure 6.31). Careful dissection is required to leave 5 to 10 mm of fasciae over the lateral and medial border of the anterior rectus sheath so as to facilitate direct repair of the donor defect. The rectus muscle divided proximally, and the connection between the superior and inferior epigastric systems are ligated. The muscle is separated easily from the posterior rectus sheath. The vascular skin territory, fasciae, and the rectus muscle are raised as one unit (Figure 6.31).

Figure 6.28 *Rectus abdominis flap. Location of musculocutaneous perforators.*

Figure 6.29 *Rectus abdominis flap. Incision for flap.*

Figure 6.30 *Rectus abdominis flap. Blood supply to flap.*

Figure 6.31 *Rectus abdominis flap. Raising of rectus muscle and anterior rectus sheath.*

Figure 6.28

Tendinous inscription

Inferior epigastric
vessels

Figure 6.29

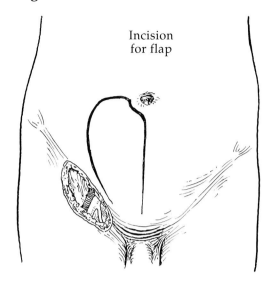

Incision
for flap

Figure 6.30

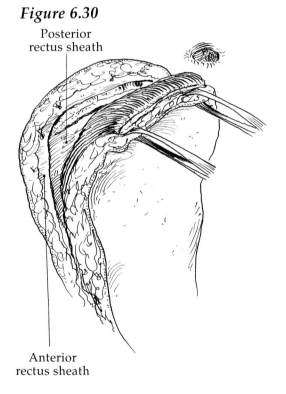

Posterior
rectus sheath

Anterior
rectus sheath

Figure 6.31

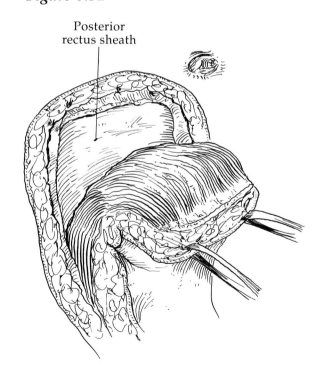

Posterior
rectus sheath

The dissection of the pedicle is done last. Identification of the inferior epigastric artery is accomplished through paramedian incision over the anterior rectus sheath. Once the vascular pedicle is isolated, transposition of the flap can be easily performed without dividing the rectus abdominis muscle from the symphysis pubis (Figure 6.32). For additional freedom, the rectus abdominis muscle can be detached and left as an island pedicle flap. Closure of the rectus abdominis fasciae is made as anatomical as possible (Figure 6.33).

Figure 6.32 *Rectus abdominis flap. Flap in place.*

Figure 6.33 *Closure of the rectus abdominis fasciae.*

Surgery for Local Tumor Recurrence of the Superficial Inguinal Region

Figure 6.32   *Figure 6.33*

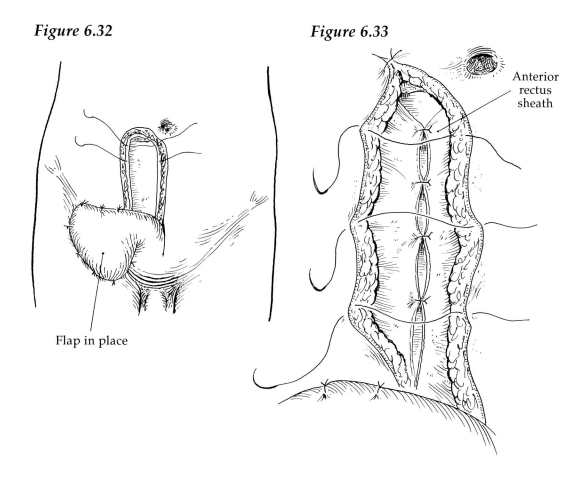

Anterior
rectus
sheath

Flap in place

Chapter 7

Reconstruction of the Urinary Tract during Surgery for Rectal Tumors

Although in the past abdominal perineal resection was the standard treatment for low rectal tumors and complete pelvic exenteration was used when these tumors invaded either the prostate or the bladder, modern surgical techniques have allowed for complete reconstruction of the gastrointestinal and urinary tract [Campbell et al., 1993; Skinner and Sherrod, 1990]. In this chapter I will describe a technique we have used for rectal tumors which are in close proximity to or invading the prostate. This approach has been used together with the assistance of a team of colorectal surgeons for complete reconstruction of the rectal and urinary tract. A long up-and-down incision is used (Figure 7.1). A complete mobilization of the sigmoid and descending colon, including the splenic flexure, is performed with ligation of the inferior mesenteric artery at the aorta (Figure 7.2). The retrorectal space is entered after the incision of the posterior peritoneal and the rectum is mobilized posteriorly (Figure 7.3). The lateral attachments of the rectum are transected (Figure 7.4). At this point attention is drawn towards the prostate, which is mobilized in the same manner as for a radical prostatectomy (Chapter 5). The puboprostatic ligaments are shown transected, the dorsal vein of the penis complex ligated, and the urethra transected (Figure 7.5). The prostate is partially mobilized from the rectum (Figure 7.6). The bladder neck is transected and the ampullae of the vas ligated (Figure 7.7). The surgical specimen, which is comprised of the sigmoid colon, rectum, prostate, and seminal vesicles, is removed en bloc (Figure 7.8). Under complete direct vision, an anastomosis between the rectal stump and the descending colon is performed. The bladder is then reanastomosed to the urethra in the same manner as in a radical prostatectomy (Chapter 5) (Figure 7.8). Care of the urinary tract is the same as for radical prostatectomy (Chapter 5).

Figure 7.1 *Reconstruction of the urinary tract. Incision.*

Figure 7.2 *Reconstruction of the urinary tract. Mobilization of the sigmoid and descending colon.*

Figure 7.3 *Reconstruction of the urinary tract. Mobilization of the rectum.*

Reconstruction of the Urinary Tract during Surgery for Rectal Tumors

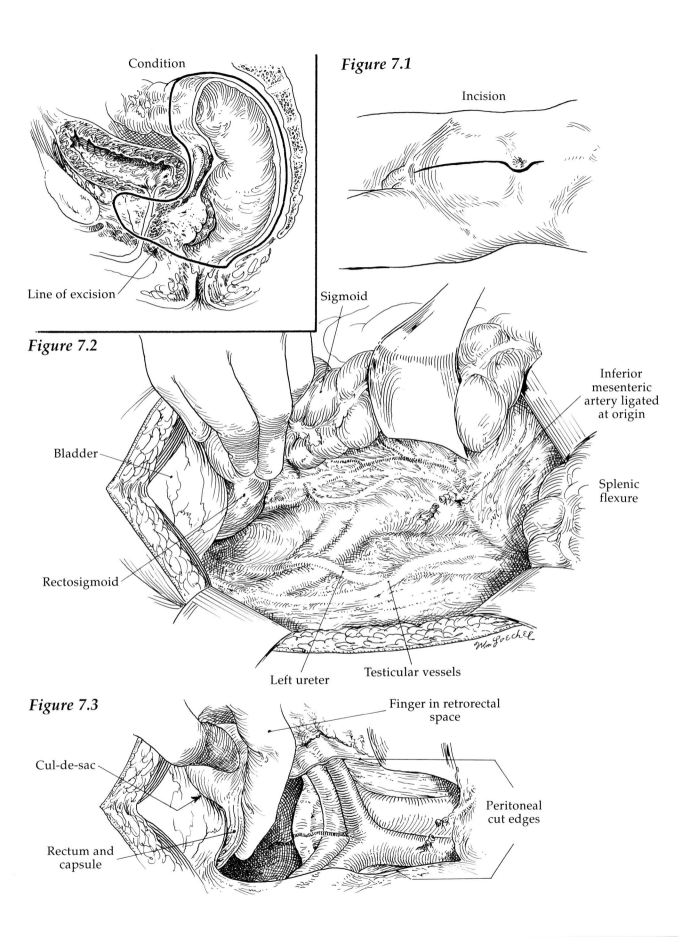

Condition

Line of excision

Figure 7.1

Incision

Sigmoid

Figure 7.2

Bladder

Rectosigmoid

Inferior
mesenteric
artery ligated
at origin

Splenic
flexure

Left ureter

Testicular vessels

Figure 7.3

Cul-de-sac

Rectum and
capsule

Finger in retrorectal
space

Peritoneal
cut edges

Reconstruction of the Urinary Tract during Surgery for Rectal Tumors

Figure 7.4   *Reconstruction of the urinary tract. Transection of the lateral attachments of the rectum.*

Figure 7.5   *Reconstruction of the urinary tract. Mobilization of the prostate.*

Figure 7.6   *Reconstruction of the urinary tract. Partial mobilization of the prostate from the rectum.*

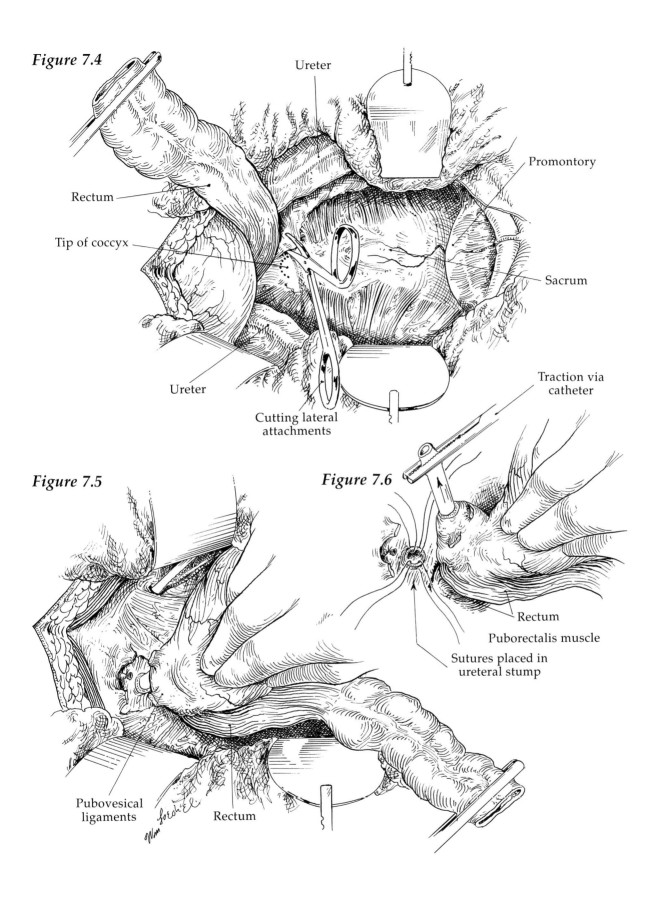

Figure 7.4

Ureter

Promontory

Rectum

Sacrum

Tip of coccyx

Ureter

Cutting lateral
attachments

Traction via
catheter

Figure 7.5

Figure 7.6

Rectum

Puborectalis muscle

Sutures placed in
ureteral stump

Pubovesical
ligaments

Rectum

Figure 7.7 *Reconstruction of the urinary tract. Transection of the bladder neck and ligation of the ampullae of the vas.*

Figure 7.8 *Reconstruction of the urinary tract. Removal of the specimen (left) is followed by anastomosis.*

Figure 7.7

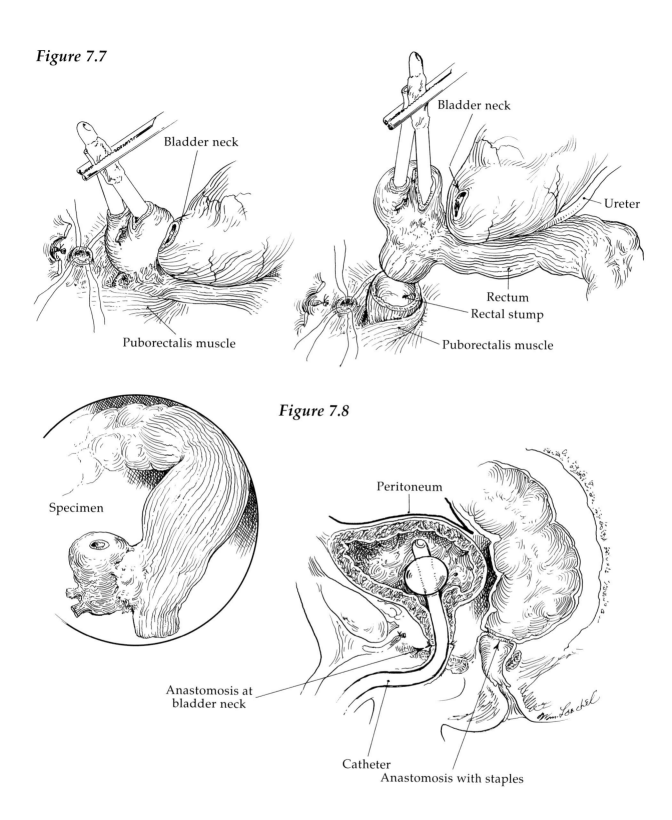

Bladder neck

Bladder neck

Ureter

Rectum

Rectal stump

Puborectalis muscle

Puborectalis muscle

Figure 7.8

Specimen

Peritoneum

Anastomosis at
bladder neck

Catheter

Anastomosis with staples

Reconstruction of the Urinary Tract during Surgery for Rectal Tumors

Chapter 8

Pelvic Sarcomas

Not uncommonly, the urological surgeon is asked to participate, as part of a team, in the management of large pelvic sarcomas. To a great extent, initial complete surgical excision of these tumors is the most important step in determining the final outcome. Using modern diagnostic techniques such as magnetic resonance imaging, with bone grafts, a large number of these tumors can be removed with restoration of musculoskeletal function. The role of the urologist in such cases is to isolate and preserve the urinary organs and to assure a tumor-free margin of the pelvic soft tissues.

An example of such a condition in this chapter is a local recurrent liposarcoma involving the obturator foramen (Figure 8.1). An outline of the area of resection is shown (Figure 8.1). The choice of incision is dictated by the extent of bone resection needed. The vertical abdominal incision shown in Figure 8.1 gives access to the soft-tissue area of the tumor. A complete exposure of the tumor is obtained by medial retraction of the bladder, right ureter, and uterus, followed by upward retraction of the bowel (Figure 8.2). The tumor involves the obturator nerve and the lateral wall muscles (Figure 8.2). The pelvic floor is shown on the left of the incision.

Figure 8.1 *Local recurrent liposarcoma of the obturator foramen* (inset). *Incisions* (right).

Figure 8.2 *Pelvic sarcoma. Complete exposure of the tumor by retraction of the bladder, right ureter, uterus, and bowel.*

Pelvic Sarcomas

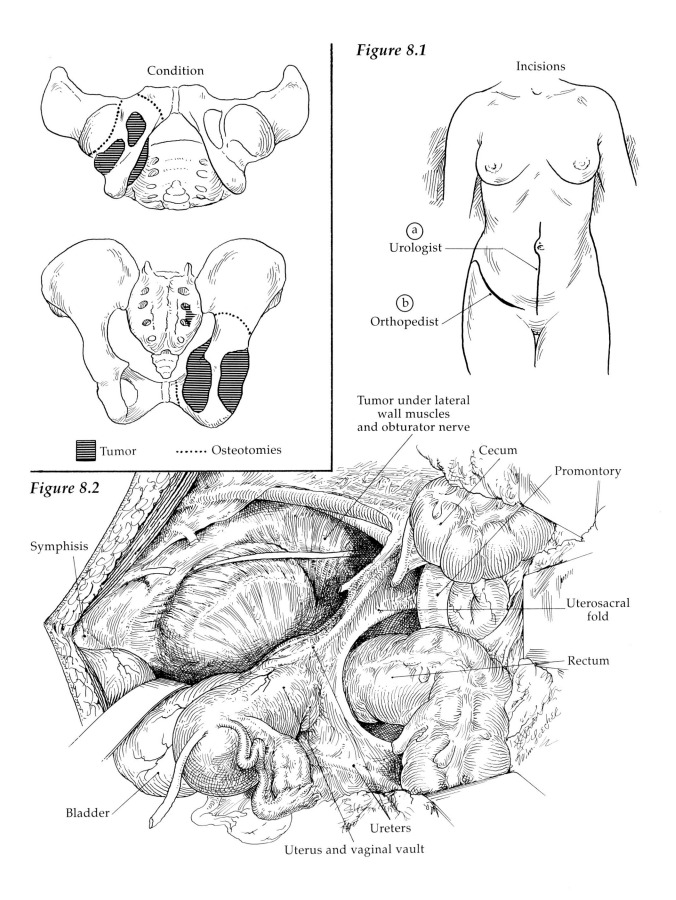

Condition

Figure 8.1

Incisions

(a) Urologist

(b) Orthopedist

■ Tumor   ⋯⋯ Osteotomies

Figure 8.2

Tumor under lateral wall muscles and obturator nerve

Cecum

Promontory

Symphisis

Uterosacral fold

Rectum

Bladder

Ureters

Uterus and vaginal vault

A wide excision of the tumor is started externally by incising the obturator internus and a portion of the levator ani (Figure 8.3). Branches of the internal iliac artery and internal pudendal vessels are ligated (Figure 8.4 inset). The muscular incision is carried medially, with partial excision of the pubococcygeus portion of the levator ani and the urogenital diaphragm (Figure 8.4). Preservation of the urethra medially, and preservation of the vagina are important as long as a negative tumor margin can be obtained (Figure 8.4).

Proceeding with a deeper resection of pelvic muscles, the iliac vessels are retracted medially and the femoral nerve is identified and isolated (Figure 8.5). Transection of the lower part of the psoas muscle and the iliacus muscle will expose the iliac bone internally (Figure 8.5). The tumor is completely isolated within the pelvic cavity and the procedure is turned over to the orthopedic team for bone resection and grafting.

Although it is not directly related to urological surgery, the orthopedic procedure is illustrated in Figure 8.6. The femur has been temporarily disarticulated, the muscle attachments of the iliac and pubic bone have been transected, and the area of the bone to be removed is outlined (Figure 8.6). After complete excision of the tumor, a bone graft is inserted with fixation (Figure 8.7), the femoral head is returned to its position, and the muscles are reattached (Figure 8.8).

These combined procedures can allow for complete removal of large pelvic tumors with excellent functional results.

Figure 8.3 *Pelvic sarcoma. Wide excision of the tumor; incision of the obturator internus and the levator ani.*

Figure 8.4 *Pelvic sarcoma. Ligation of the internal iliac artery and internal pudendal vessels (inset); partial excision of the levator ani and urogenital diaphragm.*

Pelvic Sarcomas

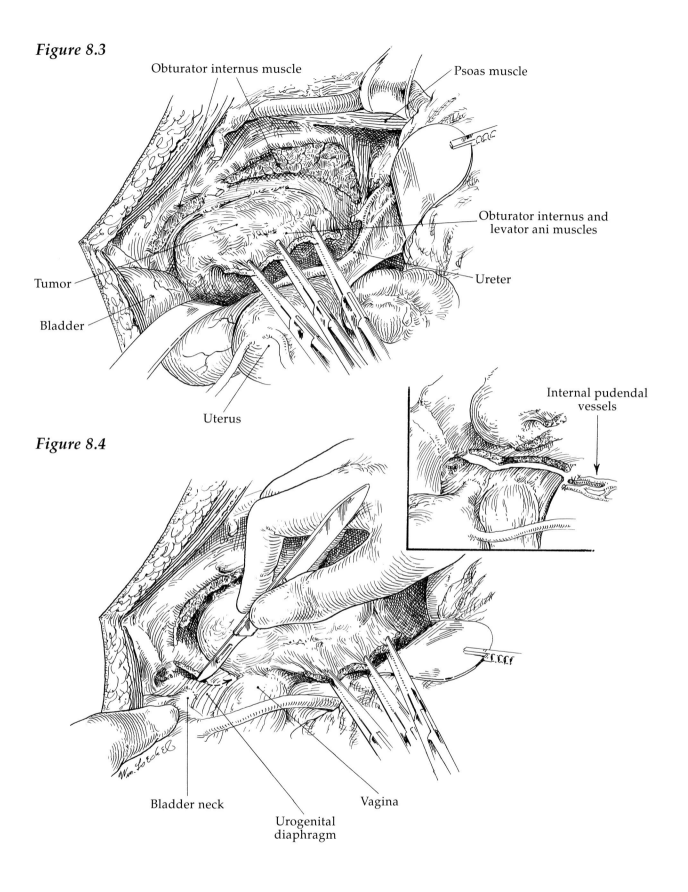

Figure 8.3

Obturator internus muscle

Psoas muscle

Obturator internus and
levator ani muscles

Ureter

Tumor

Bladder

Uterus

Figure 8.4

Internal pudendal
vessels

Bladder neck

Urogenital
diaphragm

Vagina

Figure 8.5   *Pelvic sarcoma. Deep resection of pelvic muscles to expose the iliac bone.*

Figure 8.6   *Pelvic sarcoma. Orthopedic excision.*

Figure 8.7   *Pelvic sarcoma. Bone graft with fixation.*

Figure 8.8   *Pelvic sarcoma. Repositioning of the femoral head and reattachment of the muscles.*

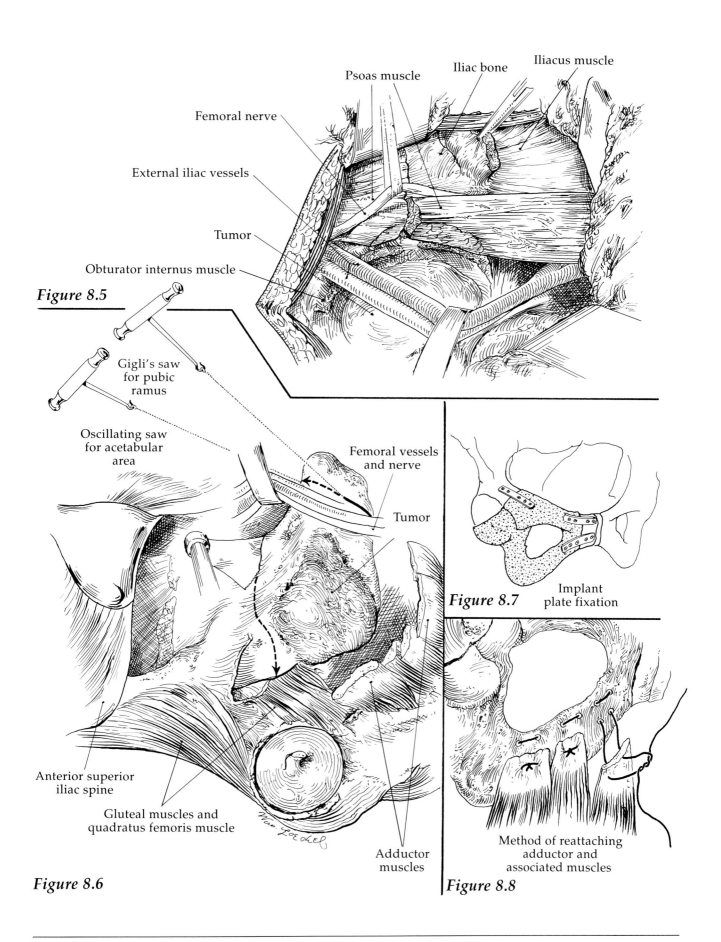

Femoral nerve

External iliac vessels

Tumor

Obturator internus muscle

Psoas muscle

Iliac bone

Iliacus muscle

Figure 8.5

Gigli's saw for pubic ramus

Oscillating saw for acetabular area

Femoral vessels and nerve

Tumor

Implant plate fixation

Figure 8.7

Anterior superior iliac spine

Gluteal muscles and quadratus femoris muscle

Adductor muscles

Method of reattaching adductor and associated muscles

Figure 8.6

Figure 8.8

References

Abi-Aad AS, DeKernion JB (1992): Controversies in ilioinguinal lymphadenectomy for cancer of the penis. Urol Clin North Am 19:319.

Bissada NK (1992): Conservative extripative treatment of cancer of the penis. Urol Clin North Am 19:283.

Campbell SC, Church JM, Fazio VW, Klein EA, Pontes JE (1993): Combined radical retropubic prostatectomy and proctosigmoidectomy for en bloc removal of locally invasive rectal carcinoma. Surg Gynecol Obstet (in press).

Gardner E, Gray DJ, O'Rahilley R (1975): "Anatomy: A Regional Study of Human Structure." Philadelphia: Saunders.

Hollinshead WH (1956): "Anatomy for Surgeons," Vol 2. New York: Harper & Brothers, pp 643–689.

LeDuc A, Camey M, Teillac P (1987): An original antireflux ureteroileal implantation technique: long-term follow-up. J Urol 137:1156.

Light JK, Engelman N (1986): LeBag: total replacement of the bladder using an ileocolonic pouch. J Urol 136:27.

Montie JE (1983): Technique of radical cystectomy. Semin Urol 1:42.

Montie JE, Pontes JE, Smyth EM (1987): Selection of the type of urinary diversion in conjunction with radical cystectomy. J Urol 137:1154.

O'Connor VJ Jr (1979): Review of experience with vesicovaginal fistula repair. Trans Am Assoc Genitourin Surg 7:120.

Pierce JM Jr (1989): Omentum in urologic surgery. In Novick AC, Streem SB, Pontes JE (eds): "Stewart's Operative Urology." Baltimore: Williams & Wilkins, p 60.

Pontes JE (1974): Rotation of bladder flap for repair of vesicovaginal fistula. Urology 4:109.

Pontes JE (1989): Radical retropubic prostatectomy. In Novick AC, Streem SB, Pontes JE (eds): "Stewart's Operative Urology." Baltimore: Williams & Wilkins, p 621.

Pontes JE (1991): Commentary: partial cystectomy. In Whitehead ED (ed): "Current Operative Urology." Philadelphia: JB Lippincott, p 176.

Pontes JE (1992): Penile cancer. Curr Opin Urol 2:369.

Rowland RG, Mitchell ME, Bihrle R, Kahnoski J, Piser JE (1987): Indiana continent urinary reservoir. J Urol 137:1136.

Skinner DG, Sherrod A (1990): Total pelvic exenteration with simultaneous bowel and urinary reconstruction. J Urol 144:1433.

Studer UE, Gerber E, Springer J, Zingg EJ (1992): Bladder reconstruction with bowel after radical cystectomy. J Urol 10:11.

Walsh PC, Lepor H, Eggleston JC (1983): Radical prostatectomy with preservation of sexual function: anatomical and pathological considerations. Prostate 4:473.

Index

Acetabular ligaments, 5
Acetabulum, 3
Ala, 3
Alcock's canal (obturator fascia), 9
Anatomy, pelvic, 1–16. *See also* Pelvic
    anatomy *and individual structures*
Anterior iliac spine, 3
Anterior longitudinal ligament, 5
Arcuate ligament, 5
Autonomic innervation of pelvis,
    10–11

Bladder: anatomy, 14–15
Bladder: surgical procedures
    cystectomy
        partial, 18–21
        partial for tumors near ureteral
            orifice, 24–25
        radical, 30–37
        radical in women, 38
    distal ureterectomy with ureteral
        reimplant, 26–27
    diverticulectomy, 22
    pelvic lymphadenectomy in bladder
        cancer, 28–29
Blood vessels of pelvis, 12–13
Bony pelvis: anatomy, 2–3
Bricker ureteroileal anastomosis, ileal
    loop, ileal conduit, 42–43

Broad ligament, 13
Bulbocavernous muscle, 15
Bulbourethral gland, 15

Coccygeus muscle, 7, 9
Cornua, 3
Cutaneous nerves, 11
Cystectomy; *see also* Diversion
    procedures
    partial, 18–21
    partial for tumors near ureteral
        orifice, 24–25
    radical, 30–37
    radical in women, 38

Denonvilliers' fascia (rectovesical
    septum)
    anatomy, 15, 16
    prostatic dissection by, 78–79
Diversion procedures
    continent
        to skin, 46–51
        to urethra: LeBag technique,
            52–53
        to urethra: W pouch technique,
            54–57
    noncontinent
        Bricker ureteroileal anastomosis,
            42–43

ileal conduit, 40–41
  Wallace ureteroileal anastomosis,
    44–45
Diverticulectomy: bladder, 22–23
Dorsal vein of the penis complex in
  radical prostatectomy, 76

Epigastric artery and vein, 13

Femoral nerve, 11
Fistulas
  vesicoenteric, 66–69
    with omentum flap, 70–71
  vesicovaginal
    abdominal repair, 62–65
    vaginal repair, 60–61
Flap procedures
  omentum, 70–71
  rectus abdominis flap, 96–99
  tensor fasciae latae flap, 94–96

Gemelli muscle, 7
Genitofemoral nerve, 11
Gluteal arteries, 13
Gluteus maximus muscle, 7

Hemorrhoidal arteries, 13
Hemorrhoidal plexuses, 11
Hypogastric plexus, 11

Ileal conduit technique, 40–41
Iliac artery and vein, 13
Iliac crest, 3
Iliac fossa, 3
Iliac spine, 3
Iliacus muscle, 7
Iliococcygeus muscle, 9
Iliofemoral ligament, 5
Iliohypogastric nerve, 11
Ilioinguinal nerve, 11
Iliolumbar ligaments, 5
Iliolumbar artery and vein, 13
Iliopectineal eminence, 3
Indiana pouch technique, 46–51
Inguinal ligament, 5
Inguinal lymph node dissection:
  superficial, 88–91
Inguinal tumor recurrence, 92–93
Inlet of pelvis, 3
Interlacunar ligament, 5
Interspinal ligament, 5
Ischial spine, 3
Ischial tuberosity, 3
Ischiocavernus muscle, 15

LeBag diversion, 52–53
LeDuc ureteral anastomosis, 46, 51, 56
Ligaments of pelvis, 3–9
Ligamentum teres femoris, 5
Longitudinal ligaments, 5
Lymphadenectomy
  pelvic in bladder cancer, 28–29
  in radical prostatectomy, 74–75
Lymph node dissection: superficial
  inguinal, 88–91

Mesenteric plexus, 11
Montie radical cystectomy technique,
  30–37
Multifidus muscle, 7
Muscles of pelvis, 3–9

Nerves of pelvis, 10–11

Obliquus internus abdominis muscle, 7
Obturator artery and vein, 13
Obturator canal, 9
Obturator fascia (Alcock's canal), 9
Obturator foramen
  anatomy, 3
  sarcoma of, 110–115
Obturator membrane, 5
Obturator muscles, 7
Omentum flap technique, 70–71
Ovaries
  anatomy, 15
  vasculature, 13, 15

Pelvic anatomy
  autonomic nervous system, 10–11
  bony pelvis, 2–3
  general features, 1
  muscles and ligaments, 3–9
  nerves and plexuses, 10–11
  urogenital organs, 14–16
Pelvic lymphadenectomy in bladder
  cancer, 28–29
Pelvic sarcoma, 110–115
  orthopedic reconstruction in,
    112–113, 115
Penectomy
  partial, 82–83
  reconstruction procedures, 94–99
  total, 84–87
Penile/urethral cancers
  flap procedures
    rectus abdominis flap, 96–99
    tensor fasciae latae flap, 94–96
  inguinal lymph node dissection:
    superficial, 88–91

local tumor recurrence of superficial
    inguinal region, 92–93
metastatic urethral carcinoma, 92–94
penectomy
    partial, 82–83
    total, 84–87
Penis
    anatomy, 15, 83
    dorsal blood vessels, 13, 16
Perineal muscles, 9
Peritoneum, 13, 15
Piriformis muscle, 7
Plexuses. *See* Nerves *and individual*
    structures
Posterior iliac spine, 3
Posterior sacroiliac ligaments, 5
Posterior superficial sacroccygeal
    ligament, 5
Promontory of pelvis, 3
Prostate
    anatomy, 15, 16
    retrograde dissection, 35, 78–79
Prostatectomy, radical, 16, 74–79
Prostatic plexus, 11
Psoas major and minor muscles, 7
Pubic ligaments, 5
Pubic tubercles, 3
Pubobulbar fibers, 9
Pubococcygeus muscle, 9, 16
Pubofemoral ligament, 5
Puboprostatic ligaments, 9, 16
Puborectalis muscle, 9
Pudendal artery, 13
Pudendal nerve, 11
Pyriformis muscle, 7

Quadratus lumborum muscle, 7

Radical cystectomy, 30–37
    in women, 38
Radical prostatectomy, 16, 74–79
Reconstruction
    postpenectomy, 94–99
    urinary tract, 102–107
Rectococcygeus muscle, 9
Rectouterine pouch, 15
Rectovesical septum (Denonvilliers'
    fascia)
    anatomy, 15, 16
    prostatic resection by, 78–79
Rectus abdominis flap, 96–99
Rectus femoris muscle, 7
Round ligament, 15

Sacral artery and vein, 13
Sacral crest, 3
Sacrococcygeal ligaments, 5
Sacroiliac ligaments, 5, 7
Sacrospinalis muscle, 7
Sacrospinous ligament, 5
Sacrotuberous ligament, 5, 9
Sarcoma, pelvic, 110–115
    orthopedic reconstruction in,
        112–113
Sartorius muscle dissection, 90–91
Sciatic notch, 3
Seminal vesicle, 15
Subcostal nerve, 11
Superior pubic ligament, 5
Supra-articular process, 3

Tensor fasciae latae flap, 94–96
Teres femoris ligament, 5
Transverse acetabular ligament, 5
Tuberosity of ilium, 3
Turnbull stoma, 44, 45

Umbilical artery, 13
Urachus, 15
Ureter: anatomy, 13, 14–15
Ureter: surgical procedures
    for bladder tumor near ureteral
        orifice, 24–25
    distal ureterectomy–ureteral
        implant, 26–27
Ureteroileal anastomosis
    Bricker technique, 42–43
    Wallace technique, 44–45
Urethra: incision in radical
    cystectomy, 35
Urethral metastasis, 92–94
Urethral/penile cancers, 82–99; *see also*
    Penile/urethral cancers
Urinary bladder. *See* Bladder
Urinary diversion. *See* Diversion
    procedures
Urinary fistulas. *See* Fistulas
Urinary tract reconstruction, 102–107
Uterine tube, 15
Uterosacral fold, 15
Uterus
    anatomy, 15
    vasculature, 13

Vagina, 15
Vascular system of pelvis, 12–13
Vas deferens, 15
Vesical arteries, 13
Vesical plexuses, 11

Vesicoenteric fistulas, 66–69
  with omentum flap, 70–71
Vesicovaginal fistulas
  abdominal repair, 62–65
  vaginal repair, 60–61

Wallace ureteroileal anastomosis,
  44–45
W pouch diversion, 54–57